CLINICAL APPLICATIONS OF MUSIC IN NEUROLOGIC REHABILITATION

Concetta M. Tomaino, ACMT-BC,
Editor

MMB

MMB MUSIC, INC.

Clinical Applications of Music in Neurologic Rehabilitation

Concetta M. Tomaino, ACMT-BC,
Editor

Cover design: Jill Wade
Typography: Bruce W. Ross
Printer: United Graphics, Mattoon, IL
1st printing: June, 1998
Printed in USA
ISBN: 1-58106-001-7

For further information and catalogs contact:

MMB Music, Inc.
Contemporary Arts Building
3526 Washington Avenue
Saint Louis, MO 63103-1019

Phone: 314-531-9635, 800-543-3771 (USA/Canada)
Fax: 314-531-8384
E-mail: mmbmusic@mmbmusic.com
Web site: http://www.mmbmusic.com

TABLE OF CONTENTS

CONTRIBUTORS

Alicia Ann Clair, Ph.D., RMT-BC, is Professor and Director of Music Therapy at the University of Kansas where she is also a Research Associate in Gerontology. Ms. Clair is Past President of the National Association for Music Therapy. She has published extensively on the applications of music therapy for persons with dementia and is nationally and internationally recognized for her research in this area.

Helen Mandel Grob, M.M., RMT-BC, CPvT., is Assistant Professor of Rehabilitation Medicine and Director of Music Therapy and Clinical Training at New York Medical College Terence Cardinal Cooke Health Care Center. In addition to her work in music therapy, Ms. Grob is a certified paraverbal therapist, master teacher and supervisor. She has published on the use of music and paraverbal techniques and is renowned for her work in this area.

Michael Hillman is a music educator and professional musician in Minneapolis, Minnesota. He received his Masters degree in Music Education at Lehman College and taught for five years at Mt. Pleasant-Blythedale UFSD. At Blythedale, he explored ways for special students to perform music in a nontraditional manner, utilizing MIDI and computers as a means of producing music on many different levels. He continues to use MIDI as an educational and performance tool.

Joseph Nagler, DA, CMT, is a music therapist, composer, and musician, who received his doctorate in music therapy at NYU. He is adjunct professor of music therapy at NYU and the Director of Research at the Center for Research in the Arts & Medicine, New York University's Rusk Institute of Rehabilitation Medicine. Additionally, he works for the New York City Board of Education as a music therapist. As a composer, Dr. Nagler has been featured on several national and international recordings for television and radio.

Oliver Sacks, M.D., was born in London and educated in London, Oxford, California, and New York. He is a clinical consultant in neurology at Beth Abraham Health Services and a cofounder of the Institute for Music and Neurologic Function. He is a Clinical Professor of Neurology at the Albert Einstein College of Medicine. Dr. Sacks lectures internationally and is the author of *Awakenings, Migraine, A Leg to Stand on, The Man who Mistook His Wife for a Hat, Seeing Voices, An Anthropologist on Mars,* and *Island of the Color Blind.*

Concetta M. Tomaino, ACMT-BC, is Director of the Department of Music Therapy at Beth Abraham Health Services. She is Past President of the American Association for Music Therapy and is a clinical music therapy supervisor at New York University where she is completing her doctoral studies. Ms. Tomaino serves on the advisory boards of the Institute for Music and Neurologic Function and the Center for Alternative Medicine Research in Rehabilitation at the Kessler Institute. She is internationally recognized for her research and music therapy work for persons with neurologic diseases.

PREFACE

The following papers are based on proceedings of the "Clinical Applications of Music in Neurologic Rehabilitation" conference sponsored by Beth Abraham Health Services in March 1993. The idea for a conference on music and neurologic function had long been a dream of mine and, after speaking to other music therapists prior to this event, realized that there was indeed a growing interest in this area of study. Since this decade has been termed the "decade of the brain", it is appropriate that efforts are made to study not only how music affects the brain but how these effects can be applied clinically to enhance the lives of those with neurologic diseases. Although the primary focus of this conference was on the "Clinical Applications of Music in Neurologic Rehabilitation" the topics ranged from the effect of music on brain function to specific technologies used to facilitate rehabilitation.

Oliver Sacks, who has written many times about music in his clinical tales, has for the first time written specifically about "Music and the Brain." Alicia Clair speaks of reaching even the most severely impaired Alzheimer's patient through music and of how this contact can allow for interactions between patient and care-giver not possible outside the music therapy session. Connie Tomaino presents examples of how music can stimulate seemingly lost motor and cognitive function through activation of alternative neural networks. Helen Grob documents responses to music, utilizing paraverbal/psychomoter techniques in rehabilitation and habilitation. Joe Nagler demonstrates how to incorporate MIDI technology in music therapy for those with limited physical ability and highlights his work with a remarkable individual. Michael Hillman introduces the "Soundbeam" and his applications of this new technology for children with special needs. In 1993, only 100 "Soundbeam" units were in use worldwide, today more than 1000 are used in a variety of clinical and educational settings.

Readers will find these papers useful from both a historical and contemporary point of view. This conference also served as the cornerstone for the annual "Music Has Power" conference series and was the foundation of the Institute for Music and Neurologic Function which was incorporated in September 1995. The Institute supports research studies related to the impact of music on learning, memory, language, hearing and recovery from nerve damage and is the sponsor of the annual "Music has Power" conference.

I would like to thank the authors for their contribution to this book and for their dedication to the advancement of music therapy. I would also like to thank William Frohlich, President of Beth Abraham Health Services, and Arnold Goldstein, Director of the Institute for Music and Neurologic Function, for their support of clinical music therapy practice and scientific research that investigates the effects of music on brain function.

Concetta M. Tomaino, ACMT-BC
Director, Department of Music Therapy
Beth Abraham Health Services, Bronx, NY

The following publishers have graciously granted permission to reproduce previously copyrighted material.

Page 20, Figure 1. Reprinted by permission, from Hodges, Donald A.., ed. *Handbook of Music Psychology*, 2d ed. San Antonio, Tex.: IMPRESS, Univ. of Texas at San Antonio, 1996, 90.

Page 21, Figure 2. Reprinted from Koepchen, et al., "Physiological Rhythmicity and Music in Medicine," in *MusicMedicine*, edited by Ralph Spintge and Roland Droh, 45. Saint Louis, Mo.: MMB Music, Inc., 1992.

FOREWORD

Much has transpired at Beth Abraham since March of 1993. I have to acknowledge that for many years I was unaware of the scope and depth of the work of music therapy. Connie Tomaino and Oliver Sacks have demonstrated to me, as an administrator, the important role music therapy plays in the lives of our residents. Our commitment to music therapy and its role in neurologic rehabilitation convinced us to move ahead with the creation of The Institute for Music and Neurologic Function. The mission of the institute is to improve the health and welfare of patients through new and more effective therapies gleaned from research and education. It engages in basic scientific research in collaboration with outstanding investigative scientists and biomedical researchers and in clinical research with physicians, music therapists, musicians and other professionals. Present areas of investigation include: Music and hearing, music and language, music and memory, music and learning and music and recovery from nerve injury. In 1994, a separate department of music therapy was created with Connie Tomaino as director. In addition to clinical work, the music therapy department has been able to expand its focus on research and has been the recipient of several major grants over the past four years. This department also provides clinical training to music therapy interns from universities in the United States, Europe and Asia.

William H. Frohlich, President,
Beth Abraham Health Services

Chapter 1

MUSIC AND THE BRAIN

Oliver Sacks, M.D.

Music is perhaps the most ancient of arts and surely the most elemental and mysterious: the terms "music" and "muse" are twins. Mystics since Plato have seen music as the closest a man can come to the direct apprehension of Creation—and a Creator. Philosophers since Pythagoras have compared it to mathematics. But one need not be a mystic or a philosopher, nor does one need to have any formal knowledge of music—nor, indeed, to be particularly "musical," to enjoy music and to respond to it at the deepest levels. That this should be so is curious, as many people have remarked, for there is no obvious adaptive "use" to music. Music has no clear relation to language or thought or any form of representation, and yet it can affect us as nothing else can, and at every level of the body and mind. Music is part of being human, and there is no human culture in which it is not highly developed and esteemed. Yet its very ubiquity may cause it to be trivialized in daily life: we switch on a radio, switch it off, hum a tune, tap our feet, find the words of an old song going through our minds, and think nothing of it. But to those who suffer or are neurologically impaired, the situation may be different. Music is no luxury to them, but a necessity, and may have a power beyond anything else to restore them to themselves, to restore them to health, at least in the precious few minutes that it lasts.

I am especially moved that this conference on music therapy is taking place at Beth Abraham today, because it was here, twenty-five years ago, that I first saw the immense powers of music, in a very special population of patients: the postencephalitic patients (whom I later wrote about in *Awakenings*) for whom this hospital, in 1920, had originally been opened.

When I came here in 1966, it was these patients who first commanded my attention. There were nearly eighty at the time; I saw them in the lobby, in the corridors, as well as on the wards, sometimes in strange postures, absolutely motionless, frozen. Some had been in this frozen state since they had entered the hospital, forty or more years before. All of them were victims of *encephalitis lethargica*, the viral sleeping sickness which had swept the world just after World War I. In 1966, there was no medication of any use to these patients—no medication, at least, for their frozenness, their parkinsonian, catatonic akinesia. And yet it was common knowledge among the nurses and others that these patients *could* move on occasion, and with an ease and grace which seemed to belie their parkinsonism. And that the most potent occasioner of such movement was, in fact, music.

Typically such patients could not *initiate* anything, and yet, sometimes, they were able to *respond*. Many would respond to a ball if it were thrown, and almost all of them tended to respond to music (at least if it were the "right" music and got them at the right moment, in the right way). Some patients could not initiate a single step but could be drawn into dancing and dance for hours, freely. Some could scarcely utter a syllable; their voices, if they could speak, lacked tone, lacked force, were almost spectral. But these patients were able to *sing*, loudly and clearly, with full vocal force and a normal range of expressiveness and tone (there is a beautiful example of this in the documentary film of *Awakenings*). Other patients could walk and talk, but only in a jerky, broken way, without continuity, without a steady tempo, and sometimes with incontinent accelerations (festinations)—with such patients, music could *modulate* the stream of movement or speech, give it the steadiness and control it so lacked. One patient, who had herself been a music teacher, said that her gait and speech had become "wooden, robotic, *unmusicked*" with her parkinsonism and that she needed to be "remusicked," to be restored to normal.

When I mentioned this once to W.H. Auden, he was fascinated; and, being a poet, at once brought up two "poetic" statements about what might be happening. He quoted an aphorism of the German poet Novalis, "Every disease is a musical problem, every cure is a musical solution," (and added "This seems to be literally true with these patients"); and a couple of lines from T.S. Eliot, "You are the music/while the music lasts."

The language of music, of articulation in time, is also used by neurologists in this regard: Parkinsonism is sometimes called a "kinetic stutter," and the normal flow of movements, by contrast, "kinetic melody."[1] This metaphor has been used by many neurologists: A.R. Luria, Henry Head, and V.M. Bechterev. Thus Head writes,

> "The complete act in its perfect form demands the mobilization in due sequence of a series of complex procedures; here the time relation ... is of fundamental importance. A want of chronological exactitude will throw the whole movement into disorder: its "kinetic melody" has been destroyed."

This is what happens in basal gangliar disease, in parkinsonism, and in many other conditions. This is what one hopes may be restored, if only transiently, if the patient is given music, can respond to it, and in so doing, get his own "music" back—the kinetic melody which has been lost, "the silent music of the body," as William Harvey called it in 1627.

---

1 Actual vocal stuttering can occur in parkinsonism, and is sometimes induced by L-DOPA. Not all stuttering, of course, has such a simple subcortical basis, but every sort of stutter, it has been known from antiquity, can be helped by music and musically cadenced forms of speech, as in recitation. Thus the severest stutterers are able to sing without stuttering, and usually to intone, orate, or recite as well—this is very striking with the country singer, Mel Tillis.

But with postencephalitic patients (who had so much the matter besides their parkinsonism), music could not only normalize their so-called disturbed kinetic melodies, their motor problems, but could sometimes awaken them from their lethargies, energize them, arouse them into a state of animation, of generalized "readiness." Such arousals, in themselves, had no special mental content, intentionality or emotion—but they *prepared* the nervous system for all of these. As we saw later, when we were able to make EEG studies on these patients, such arousals could effect a real physiological transformation. Many of these patients had exceedingly slow EEGs, dominated by slow waves in the 1–4 hz. (delta) range; if we could find music that worked, their EEGs would change, normalize, in the same moment as their clinical states. We observed this when patients listened to music or sang or played it—or even imagined it. One patient, Rosalie B., tended to remain transfixed for hours a day, completely motionless, stuck, usually with one finger on her spectacles. She could, however, play the piano beautifully and for hours—and when she played, her parkinsonism disappeared, giving way to ease and fluency and normality. Music liberated her from her parkinsonism for a time—and not only music, but *imagining* music. Rosalie knew all Chopin by heart, and we had only to say "Opus 49" to her to see her whole body, posture, and expression change. Her parkinsonism would vanish as the F-minor *Fantasie* played itself in her mind. The power of music to animate and organize brain activity, Kant called it "the quickening art," is particularly spectacular in patients who lack the normal ongoing motor and motor-regulatory activity the rest of us have. Music is not a luxury but a *necessity* to such patients and can (if it works, and for a while) provide what their brain can no longer supply.[2]

I say, "if it works," because, quite frequently, with such patients, music does not work. "The arts are not drugs," as E.M. Forster wrote, "they are not guaranteed to act when taken." Nor is there any such thing as "generic" music with a general action like, for example, light or photic stimulation. Thus Rosalie B. would not respond to Bach or Bartok, but only to Chopin and Schubert, the Romantics. These called to her, roused in her a special feeling and resonance.

Nietzsche was intensely interested throughout his life in the relationship of art, especially music, to physiology and bodily function. Analyzing the effects of music, he spoke, first, of its "tonic" effect—its power of arousing the nervous system in a general way, especially in states of physiological and psychological depression (he was himself often depressed, physiologically and psychologically, by severe migraines).

---

[2] The effect of music, in contrast to the effects of L-DOPA or other drugs, is virtually instantaneous: the patient suddenly switches from one neural mode to another and may do so within a fraction of a second. It is not imaginable that the chemical status of the basal ganglia could be normalized in so short a time; one must suspect, rather, that the basal ganglia are being bypassed, and that alternative neural pathways are being brought into use.

Secondly, he spoke of the "dynamic" powers of music (we now speak of its "propulsive" powers)—its ability to elicit, to drive, and to regulate movement. He especially associated the dynamic power of music with its rhythmic force, which he saw as the most primitive and powerful aspect of music.[3] Rhythm, he felt, could propel and articulate the stream of movement (and the stream of emotion and mind, that he saw as no less dynamic or motoric than the purely muscular). Rhythmic vitality, exuberance, he felt, expressed itself most naturally in the form of dance. (He called his own thinking, philosophizing, "dancing in chains," and thought the strongly rhythmic music of Bizet as ideally suited to this. He would always take his notebook to Bizet concerts and wrote, "Bizet makes me a better philosopher.")

But, of course, it was not just the rhythmic force of Bizet that appealed to him, but something more particular and personal, so that he was not just driven, propelled by it, but responded creatively to it. It is this which Forster speaks of when he says that the arts do not act in a mechanical way, but rather that "something as mysterious and capricious as the creative impulse has to be released before they can act." This complex, mysterious and capricious "something" Nietzsche called "mnemonic"—he felt this was not mediated by some relatively simple part of the brain but called to the whole individual, the "I," to the particularity of the individual's memories, associations, emotions.[4]

I had read Nietzsche's notes on *Physiology and Art* as a student many years before, but his concise and brilliant formulations came alive for me only when I came to Beth Abraham and saw the extraordinary powers of music with our postencephalitic patients—its power to "awaken" them at every level: to alertness when they were lethargic, to normal movement when they were frozen, and most uncannily, to vivid emotions and memories, fantasies, whole identities (for the most part unavailable to them). Music did everything L-DOPA, still in the future, was subsequently to do—and more; but only for the brief span it lasted, and perhaps for a few minutes, or at most hours, afterwards. But its special impact was remembered and sought and used by us all, before L-DOPA became available, and, subsequently, when the effects of medication became compromised and undependable.

---

3 Nietzsche also wrote about "the pathological" in music, which he equated with "degeneration of the sense of rhythm," and its result: shapeless melody, "the polypus in music," a development he sometimes ascribed to Wagner.

4 Schopenhauer was also extremely musical and extremely interested in the power of music; in *The World as Will and Representation,* he took music to be "pure Will." No one describes the powers of music more beautifully than Schopenhauer, although his speculations on the mechanism of its action are, unlike Nietzsche's, oddly mechanical and superficial:

> "The effects of music on the mind, so penetrating, so immediate, so unfailing, and also the aftereffect that sometimes follows it, consisting in a specially sublime frame of mind, are explained by the *passive* nature of hearing. ... The vibrations of the tones following in combined, rational, numerical relations, set the brainfibres themselves vibrating in a similar way."

It was parkinsonism, and especially the postencephalitics, which first drew my attention to the varied effects of music on the nervous system, the emotions, the mind. I should say, my *clinical* attention, for I had all sorts of personal experiences with music: finding myself calmed by it, excited by it, comforted by it, mystified by it, and often haunted by it. A friend of mine, Jonathan Miller, once called music "orange juice for the ear," and I needed it to arouse me, to start the day; needed to have it as background when I worked; liked to have it, as company, when I drove; enjoyed it, propulsively, when I went for runs and walks; and needed it, finally, to still my thoughts when I retired, to usher me into the world of dreams. Without being terribly "musical" (I could not, like my father, return from a concert, reproduce everything I had heard by ear, improvise with it, play it in different styles and keys), I found music indispensable to many aspects of my life, the intellectual no less than the emotional and physical.

But it was only in 1974, when I became a patient myself, and (like my parkinsonian patients, although my condition was different) felt myself "unmusicked," that I experienced the need for music and what it meant to be "remusicked" in an unforgettable and overwhelming way. (I describe this in my book *A Leg to Stand On.*) I had had a bad fall mountain climbing and was incapacitated by neural and muscular damage to one leg. After being rescued, I came to surgery, had the torn tendons in the leg repaired, and awaited some return of function in the torn nerves. With the leg immobilized, and effectively paralyzed, I lost all sense of its existence—I seemed to lose, indeed, the *idea* of moving it and could no longer evoke even an image of walking (such imagery is always accompanied by minute muscular movements, the movements that normally go with the action; and, if these movements are unavailable, the inner imagery is undermined). Mental effort, or "will," is useless in these circumstances, because it has no point of application. The leg stayed nonfunctional, effectively denervated, for fifteen days, the longest fifteen days of my life, and days made longer, grimmer because there was no source of music in the hospital (interference prevented radio reception), and I did not have a tape recorder, until, finally, a friend—the "orange juice" one—brought me one, with a single cassette, the Mendelssohn *Violin Concerto.* Playing this repeatedly gave me great pleasure and a general sense of being alive and well. There was, however, no specificity in the feeling: I could not translate it directly to the leg, the limb which so needed to be "remusicked." Nietzsche writes, "One listens to music with one's muscles," but I could not respond to music fully: the leg would not keep time, until its muscles (and their nerve supply) were sufficiently recovered. This took two weeks. On the fifteenth day, I was stood up to walk, but I could not, had no idea how to, until music came to my aid—*made* me do it: this coincided with the sudden playing of the *Violin Concerto*, fortissimo, in my mind. Suddenly, without thinking, I found myself walking, easily, unselfconsciously, joyfully, *with* the music. It was as if I suddenly remembered how to walk, indeed, not "as if"—*I remembered how to walk.* All of a sudden I remembered walking's natural, unconscious rhythm and melody; it came to me suddenly, like remembering a once-familiar but long forgotten tune, and it came hand in hand with the Mendelssohn rhythm and tune.

After my own leg experience, I had occasion to study many other patients with peripheral or spinal injuries, who, despite reasonable recovery, in anatomical terms, had been unable to achieve a return of body image and kinetic melody, a return of ongoing neurological function, of *use*. One such patient was an old lady with an apparently paralyzed and useless left leg. It had been like this since a complex hip fracture, followed by surgery and weeks in a cast. Surgery had been successful, but, strangely, her leg remained inert and useless. The muscles of the leg, indeed, showed a complete "electrical silence"; and evoked potential studies in the brain showed that it was no longer represented in the sensory areas—it had completely dropped out of body image. And yet there was no residual injury. Had the leg ever moved since the injury, we asked her? Yes, she said, it had: it once kept time at a Christmas concert, when an Irish jig was being played. This showed that, if there were the right musical stimulus, the leg *could* respond and move. Ordinary physiotherapy had been useless, and we wondered if music therapy could accomplish what physiotherapy had failed to do. It did. We were able to elicit strong automatic ("entrained") responses to music and rhythm, to get the patient to make dancing movements, and finally, to walk.

I think that music for her, as for me, provided a sort of template or pattern around which the movements of walking could be reorganized and centered. It helped to reorganize, or recreate, motor programs or engrams (or allow access to them) necessary for the recovery or reconstruction of what one might call the motor identity. This seemed to me rather similar to the motor organizing effects of music in parkinsonians—they too, listening to music (if there is a point at which music is effective) suddenly "remember" how to walk or move in a nonparkinsonian way, how to move from a parkinsonian to a normal identity, just as they do when L-DOPA takes effect.

Parkinsonism, basal gangliar disorders, are disorders of *time*, disorders in the temporal organization of movement. Gerald Edelman, in *Bright Air, Brilliant Fire*, speaks of the basal ganglia as "organs of succession," and they indeed play a crucial role in organizing the temporal aspects of movement, the very aspects which Head called their "kinetic melody." My impression, speculatively, is that such templating and programming is chiefly subcortical, mediated especially by the basal ganglia (not in isolation, of course, but in their reciprocal relationships with sensory and motor regions of the cortex). I do not think that consciousness or emotion are necessarily involved at this level, nor personal memories or images or experiences.[5] Perhaps one should speak of "motor" memories at this level, or of "procedural" memories. When these are impaired,

[5] There is some suggestion that music may have some effect even in states of coma, sometimes as a visible "keeping time" with the music, sometimes as an arousal response on EEG. Patients sometimes seem to have memories of music that was played when they were in coma, and it is sometimes suggested that music stimulation may actually shorten coma (though it is very difficult to know how one might verify this). Nevertheless, it may be worth providing such patients with music in the environment, however faint the possibility of a therapeutic reaction.

as they are in parkinsonism and other basal gangliar disorders, music can act as a sort of temporary substitute, a "prosthesis" for the basal ganglia, in particular of its functions as a temporal organizer and sequencer of movement.

This may be so at even more primitive levels, such as that of the cerebellar regulation of movement. Thus, it has been observed that music may temporarily restore coordination in those who have become incoordinate from alcohol. A colleague, Dr. Richard Garrison, describes this in a recent letter, regarding a group of older people at a party:

> "As they drank heavily, and the clock approached midnight, they became progressively more ataxic between tunes. As they would become drunker, and stagger between each [number], their dancing seemed *unaffected*. ... One gentleman would spring out of his chair every time we started playing, then collapse after we quit. He seemed unable to walk onto the dance floor, but rather danced his way out."

Patients with cerebellar damage (or any of us if we are drunk) have a sense of uncontrol, that our movements and muscles have escaped from us, from our will. Parkinsonian patients and patients with other basal gangliar disorders (chorea, dystonias, dyskinesias, etc.) have a somewhat different sense, a sense rather of being puppets—controlled by a low-order "will" not truly their own. Thus, the forced hurrying or festination of the parkinsonian is experienced as both passive and compulsive: *he* is not walking, moving, of his own volition, but *being* walked, rushed, by a force not his own. This is precisely what Gaubius expressed, writing of festination ("scelotyrbe festinans") almost a century before Parkinson: "Cases occur in which the muscles, duly excited by the impulses of the will, do then, with an unbidden agility, and with an impetus not to be repressed, run before the unwilling mind."[6]

Yet music, in such patients, must be seen as operating not only as a subcortical prosthesis, but as calling upon the active powers of the self, the motor identity—the "will"—stimulating it to reappropriate motor control. (Schopenhauer, in *The World as Will and Representation*, sees music as "pure will.")

A different and far more complex form of movement disorder and, indeed, action disorder is to be seen in Tourette's syndrome, where there may be violent, convulsive tics and uncoordinate, explosive movements of all sorts, as well as incontinent motor reactions to inner and outer stimuli—a state not merely demusicked, but *decentered*. And yet, even in the severest cases of Tourette's syndrome, the effects of music, when attended to, or especially if performed, can be little short of incredible. I saw this spectacularly in a severely affected patient who seemed almost dispossessed, at times, by the violence of his Tourette's. But this man, so frenetic for most of the time, could play the guitar and sing; and, when he did this, he came together completely, was freed of his explosive tics and impulses, restored to himself. As soon as the music ended, he would disintegrate once again. There was no tension, no suppression of his tics

---

[6] Patients with basal gangliar disorders, and also with myclonic and tic disorders, can also be driven deeper into their disorders by music, if it is the "wrong" sort of music—perhaps overloud music, or over-forceful rhythms, which may cause them to jump or jerk with the beat, like marionettes or mechanical dolls.

with concentration, but rather a different neural or psychic mode, an integration of his usually shattered nervous system and being, an achievement, albeit temporary, of a deep functional unity.

David Aldridge, a jazz drummer with Tourette's, has written of himself in "Rhythm Man": "Jazz ... soothed my Tourette syndrome like nothing I'd ever experienced." And yet this was not so much a suppression or loss of Tourette's, as a use of it, a control of it, in a musical, personal way. "Rhythm and Tourette syndrome have been intertwined," Aldridge writes, "from the first day that I found that drumming on a table could mask my jerky hand, leg and neck movement ... could harness my unbounding (Tourettic) energy, direct it into an orderly flow." He describes how, with jazz, the "roller-coaster ride" of Tourette's could be transformed, because he was riding it, controlling it, not it him.[7]

Such descriptions sharpen for us Nietzsche's concept of the "dynamic" in relation to music, especially rhythm: it is not just a matter of motion and time, but of inner force and energy, of intention and impulse. And it is these inner characteristics which make it wholly different from a mere pacemaker or metronome—it is the inner life, the "will," of rhythm that has such power and that calls to the "will" of the performer.

Many other sorts of patients may respond powerfully and specifically to music (and sometimes, to nothing else); and for these, too, music therapy, a musical atmosphere, is essential. At a hospital like Beth Abraham, with its hundreds of chronic neurological patients, roughly one quarter of the population has parkinsonism, one quarter dementia, one quarter has suffered strokes, and the remaining quarter has a whole range of problems from multiple sclerosis to spinal tumors, cerebral palsy to cerebral trauma. Some of these patients have diffuse cortical disease, whether from Alzheimer's, repeated small strokes, or other causes of dementia; others have specific cortical syndromes—loss of language functions, aphasias, agnosias, apraxias, frontal-lobe syndromes, or amnestic syndromes of various sorts. All of these potentially may respond to music and music therapy.

It has been known since the first descriptions of aphasia a century and a half ago that though language may be lost or severely compromised, musical ability, and ability to play or sing, is usually preserved. Further, if an aphasic patient sings a song, some or all of its words can often be retrieved with the tune, can be carried by it, and are not wholly lost. Thus music can give *access* to

---

7 Thus there are, clearly, at least two modes of interaction between the Tourettic brain and music: first, the apparent disappearance of impulsiveness and Tourettism with the more compelling mood or mode of the music; and second, the *fusing* of the Tourettism with the music, to produce an amalgam—musicalized Tourette's (another jazz drummer I know often tics in 5/4 time), or Tourettized music, (for example, music with Tourettic exaggerations of rhythm and emphasis). One eminent composer and conductor I know of has Tourette's syndrome, but in the course of a concert at Carnegie Hall, there was not a single tic in three hours; on the other hand, in some of the grand, bravura passages in his works, there is an energy, there are sudden emphases, sudden tensions and releases, such as might make one wonder if he is not, on occasion, making creative use of his Tourette's.

language when it can no longer be accessed directly. This ability to sing words, even if one cannot speak them, invariably gives pleasure, and a sense that one is not so devastatingly disabled.

The next question is whether words embedded in a song can be disembedded and returned for ordinary speaking use. Opinions are divided here, not least because there is so much variation between patients, but there are some patients, without doubt, who can be reminded, as it were, of words and grammatical constructions they have "forgotten." With reintroduction to these, at first in a song, these patients may start to regain the old paths of access or to build new ones in their place. Music is especially valuable here as a crucial first step, in opening a door or initiating a sequence that may then be amenable to spontaneous improvement and speech therapy.

We have patients at Beth Abraham with frontal lobe damage, some of whom are apraxic and have lost the ability to carry out a complex chain of actions: to dress, for example. Here, music can be very useful as a mnemonic, or a narrative—in effect a series of commands or promptings in the form of rhyme or song, as in the childhood rhyme, "one, two, buckle my shoe." It is similar with severely retarded people, unable to perform fairly simple tasks involving perhaps four or five movements or procedures in sequence, who are enabled to do these perfectly well if they work to music. Music has the power to embed sequences and to do this when other forms of organization (including verbal forms) fail.[8]

A similar use of music, as instruction, is sometimes possible in patients with sensory agnosias, like the agnosic musician who mistook his wife for a hat. Here, too, the needs and tasks of the day could not be done directly, but only if organized in song. His wife explained to me:

> "I put all his usual clothes out, in all the usual places, and he dresses without difficulty, singing to himself. He does everything singing to himself. But if he is interrupted and loses the thread, he comes to a complete stop, doesn't know his clothes—or his own body. He sings all the time—eating songs, dressing songs, bathing songs, everything. He can't do anything unless he makes it a song."

A fascinating area—one which has especially engaged Connie Tomaino and myself—is the relation of music to memory. We have especially explored this with a young man, Greg F., who came to Beth Abraham in 1975, with a benign but massive brain tumor causing blindness, damage to his frontal lobes, and damage to the memory systems of the temporal lobes. He was an amnesiac, unable to remember anything for more than thirty seconds, and with a retrograde amnesia going back to the late 1960s. But he had extremely detailed, indeed encyclopedic, memories from before this time—that is, of his early and midteens, and of the Grateful Dead and their music, of which he was a passionate

---

[8] This power of music to embed nonmusical sequences may reach extraordinary heights in the musically gifted. Thus, Ernst Toch, the composer (his grandson Lawrence Weschler tells me), could readily hold in his mind after a single hearing a very long string of numbers; but he did this by converting the string of numbers to a tune (a melody he shaped "corresponding" to the numbers).

devotee. When one talked to Greg, the 60s came alive—they seemed vividly present to him, not (as for the rest of us) a time one had lived through and left, and which was now in the past.

Greg was still in the 60s, in effect—the 70s for him were still in the future. I was able, through the courtesy of Mickey Hart, to bring Greg to a Grateful Dead concert in September 1991. He loved the drive to New York, the smell of hot pretzels, the roar of the crowd in Madison Square Garden, the smell of marijuana there—all this was his world, the world he had never left.

In the first part of the concert, the Dead played mostly their earlier music—Greg loved this, sang along, and, at this point, was so organized, so "with it," I forgot he was a patient. But later the band went on to play some more recent songs, and then Greg became confused. "What is this?" he kept asking. "Man, it's weird stuff. I never heard anything like it. Sounds like the music of the future." This, for him, was quite literally so, because for him, in his amnesia, the 1970s and 1980s and their music had not happened, were indeed the future.

The next day, Greg had no memory of the concert, no memory that he had been taken out the previous evening—and yet, when I played him some of the "new" music, which he had heard for the first time at the concert, he was able to recognize some of it, sing along with it. This bewildered him, because the music was unusual, he thought, and he did not know where or how he could have learned it. This raised a very interesting point, which may have relevance in other conditions. Greg had lost memory of the particular scene, the context, the concert—he had no memory of this, no "episodic" memory—and yet he retained some of the music that was performed there. It seemed that a different memory system must be involved. And this, in turn, made us wonder whether one could use this system, seemingly still fairly intact despite his massive brain damage and his episodic amnesia, to serve as a matrix or framework for embedding new factual memories—memories which, in the ordinary way, he could not retain.

It is easy to show that simple information can be embedded in songs; thus, we can give Greg the date every day, in the form of a jingle, and he can readily isolate this, and say it when asked, without the jingle. But what does it mean to say, "This is July 9, 1995," when one is sunk in the profoundest amnesia, when one has lost a sense of time and history, when one is existing from moment to moment in a sequenceless limbo? Knowing the date means nothing in these circumstances. Could one, however, through the evocativeness and power of music, perhaps using songs with specially written lyrics—songs which relate something valuable about himself or the current world—accomplish something more lasting, deeper? Give Greg not only "facts," but a sense of time and history, of the relatedness of events, an entire (if artificial) framework for thinking—a musical equivalent of the classical memory systems, the *Ars Memoriae* of antiquity?

After dealing with so many specific cerebral syndromes, we need to address the powers of music with diffuse cerebral damage, with those states of disorientation and dementia which occur with advancing Alzheimer's disease, or with insults to the cortex from repeated small strokes—states which used to be called, twenty years ago, "senility." As life expectancy increases, we now see increasing numbers of such patients in nursing homes and hospitals—this may be the awful price we pay for longevity, unless we can find ways of averting such brain changes.

Nothing is more horrifying or more indicative of therapeutic futility, as well as callousness, than the all-too-common sight of dozens of demented patients, agitated and confused, tied up (for this is what "restraint" means), drugged, bereft of stimulation, ignored, shouting and banging with all their might, reduced to a subcortical level, to primitive stereotypies of the sort one sees sometimes in zoos, with large animals imprisoned in small cages. Now we are more enlightened, we are beginning to change our zoos—we know that animals need space, order, and stimulation; we now think in terms of "habitats," not cages; and, where the stimulation of nature is unavoidably deficient, we can devise others that will keep the animals from a lethal boredom. And yet, one may still visit chronic hospitals and nursing homes and see treatment one would not accord any animal, treatment that denies that these are human beings, that they have dignity, that they are capable of response. This too, happily, is beginning to change—and not least through the recognition, in the last few years, that even in deeply demented and confused patients, organization and orientation and calm may be brought about by arts and activities that have meaning and feeling. Space, beauty, and gardens are essential; cooking, gardening, and familiar activities; outings, excursions, and a sense of the real world; visits, visitors, and the world coming to them; discussion, reminiscence, poetry, and theater—at least when verbal abilities are still present; and, most crucially, even when they are not, the nonverbal powers of art, above all music. Even when dementias are far advanced, a quality and dignity of life can be nourished or restored; and nothing is more important here, in addition to everything else, than the provision of music as therapy. Indeed, even in the inhuman, impersonal terms of "cost-benefit," the benefit immeasurably exceeds the cost; and at the human, moral level, the difference is absolute, between a purely medical, largely pharmacological approach to such patients, a medicine aimed at their pathology and deficits, and one that addresses their still very real capabilities.

In dementias, one may find all sorts of specific losses—of language, of visual recognition, of executive ability, of emotional response, of memory, of thinking power, of judgement—such as we have described in other conditions; and, as the disease worsens, a reduction of personal identity. And yet this reduction is virtually never complete; it is as if identity has such a robust, widespread neural basis; as if personal style is so deeply ingrained in the nervous system that it is never wholly lost, at least while there is still any mental life present at all. (This, indeed, is what one might expect if the personal quality of experience and feeling and thought has molded the structure of the brain from the start.) And it is this that makes a continuing possibility of being affected by music, even in the most deeply damaged patients, long inaccessible to language and most other modes of communication. For it is the inner life of music that can still make contact with their inner lives, with *them*; that can awaken the hidden, seemingly extinguished soul; and evoke a wholly personal response of memory, associations, feelings, images, a return of thought and sensibility, an answering identity. Familiar music acts as a sort of Proustian mnemonic, eliciting emotions and associations that had been long forgotten, giving the patient access once again to moods and memories, thoughts, and worlds that seemingly had been completely lost. One sees that there is not so much an actual loss of memories here, but a loss of access to these—music, here, can provide a key for opening the door to the past, a door not only to specific moods and memories but also to the entire thought structure and personality of the past.

That this can occur depends on the striking fact that musical memory in Alzheimer's disease (as in the amnesias) is relatively preserved, not only for recognizing music but also for performing it (if this had been possible before.) Thus a correspondent recently wrote to me:

> "Although my wife has Alzheimer's—diagnosed at least seven years ago—the essential person miraculously remains. ... She plays piano several hours daily, very well. Her present ambition is to *memorize* the Schumann A minor piano concerto."

And yet this is a woman who is, in most other spheres, grossly forgetful and disabled. (Nietzsche himself continued to improvise at the piano, long after he had been rendered mute, aphasic, demented, and partially paralyzed by tertiary syphilis.)[9]

It is not, of course, only known or familiar music that has power to evoke powerful emotions and associations, moods, modes of being, whole inner worlds. Music never heard before can have this effect too, can take one by storm, fill the mind with wonder or excitement and this is true of the demented, the amnesic, the neurologically-disabled, no less than it is of the rest of us, of us all. When music 'works', be it old or new, it serves as a communication, an intercourse, at once intimate and profound, more so than any verbal communion (which, in such patients, may in any case be impossible).

With music, the demented patient may be enabled to recall and reaccess not only his powers of speech, perceptual and thinking skills, but his entire emotional and intellectual configuration, his life history, his identity—at least for a little while. It is very poignant to see such recalls, such restorations of the otherwise lost persona. And such restorations, like the brief "awakenings" of postencephalitic patients through music, may be accompanied by striking changes in the EEG.

---

9 The extraordinary neural robustness of music—not only musical memory, but musical intelligence, musical sensibility, musicality generally—is also brought out in the following letter I recently received, about a famous pianist, now aging:

> "[He] is 88 now and has lost language ... but he plays every day. When we read through Mozart, he points back and ahead well in advance of the repeats. Two years ago we recorded the complete four-hand repertoire of Mozart that he had recorded ... in the 1950s. While his language has begun to fail him, I love his recent playing and conception even more than the earlier recording."

Especially moving here is not merely the preservation, but the apparent heightening of musical powers and sensitivity, as other powers wane. My correspondent concludes: "The extremes of musical accomplishment and illness are so plainly evident in his case; a visit be comes miraculous as he transcends the disease with music."

If such responses show us how deep and wide and robust is the neural representation of personality or identity, they show that the same is true for music, too. There are undoubtedly particular areas of the cortex subserving musical intelligence and sensibility, and there can be forms of "amusia" with damage to these.[10] But the response to music, it would seem, is widespread and probably not only cortical but subcortical, so that even in a diffuse cortical disease like Alzheimer's, music can still be perceived, enjoyed, and responded to. Where there is human consciousness, there can be a response to music; and it may be, too, that there can be responses even when there is not, for example in patients who are in coma (the period of coma, some reports seem to indicate, can be lessened by music).

Whatever other effects it may have, the primary impact of music is emotional, however complex or abstract its structure may be.[11] We see this most startlingly in patients who show the severest compromises in their emotional responses, whether due to neurotic or psychotic problems, or to organic ones. One of the earliest descriptions of the therapeutic power of music is the beautiful description in the Bible of David playing his harp to the mad Saul, restoring him to himself, to reality.[12]

---

10 It has been shown that "naive" listeners use chiefly the right hemisphere when listening to music, while sophisticated ones use their left hemispheres predominantly. A.R. Luria has provided case reports (especially striking since these often involved professional musicians) showing how a left-hemisphere lesion can cause loss of musical "intelligence," analytical musical ability, while leaving intact an emotional sensibility to music; and how a right-hemisphere lesion, by contrast, may abolish this, but leave intact formal musical intelligence.

And Otto Creutzfeldt has shown, recording neuronal activity from the exposed brain at surgery, that neurons in the lateral temporal lobe show strong responses to some aspects of musical stimuli—but he also stresses that other (and essential) responses are mediated elsewhere, or perhaps globally, in the brain.

11 This, of course, has always been recognized and was a subject of practical exploration by the Greeks with their invention of musical "modes"—Doric, Lydian, Phrygian, etc. Since the establishment of a well-tempered pitch, our scales have become symmetrical and indistinguishable—there is nothing "Effy" about F, "B-flatty" about B-flat (except, perhaps, to someone with absolute pitch). But the ancient modes are not like scales: they are instantly distinguishable in character and quality: they affect the nervous system in quite different ways. This was well understood by the Greeks and is being rediscovered now, being made the subject of new, physiological investigations. There is some suggestion of transcultural and biological universals here, the ability of these modes to "tune" the nervous system, or modify it, irrespective of culture and age. Music therapy has yet to make fuller use of these.

12 A moving description of the "cure" of a psychosis by, music is provided by Schreber in his *Memoirs of my Nervous Illness*: "During piano playing the nonsensical twaddle of the voices which talk to me is drowned. ... Every attempt at 'representing' me by the 'creation of a false feeling' and suchlike is doomed to end in failure because of the real feeling one can put into piano-playing."

Normal responses to music may still be seen even in the most regressed, dilapidated schizophrenics who have spent a lifetime institutionalized. Thus the *Register of Lunatics* for Sunnyside Royal Hospital in Scotland, in its notes on an inmate, Martha Wallace, records that, on the 1st of June, 1828, though

> "... far advanced in years ... and forty-four years in the Asylum, without any variation in the state of her mind during the whole of that time ... her susceptibility to music was evinced when on Saturday ... rising from her seat, and with a cheerful countenance, she hobbled and danced to the utmost of her strength to the sprightly tune called Neil Gow by a fiddler."

My own experience has been especially with the power of music in the profound organic affective disorders that may go with frontal lobe damage. One such patient at Beth Abraham, Harry S.—a gifted man, a former engineer—suffered a huge cerebral hemorrhage from a burst aneurysm, with gross destruction of both frontal lobes. Emerging from a coma, he started to recover, and recovered most of his formal intellectual powers, but he remained severely impaired, bland, flat, and indifferent emotionally. He would read the daily papers conscientiously, take in everything, but with an uncaring, indifferent eye. Surrounded by all the emotions, the drama, of others in the hospital—people agitated, distressed, or in pain; or, rarely, laughing and joyful—surrounded by their wishes, fears, hopes, aspirations, accidents, tragedies and occasional jubilations; he himself remained entirely unmoved, seemingly incapable of any human feeling.[13]

But all this changes, suddenly, when he sings. He has a fine tenor voice and loves Irish songs. When he sings, he does so with a fullness of feeling, a tenderness, a lyricism, that is astounding—the more so because one sees no hint of this at any other time and might well think his emotional capacity entirely destroyed. He shows every emotion appropriate to what he sings—the frivolous, the jovial, the tragic, the sublime—and seems to be transformed while he sings. How is this possible without frontal lobes? It is as if the songs enable him to retrieve emotions to which he otherwise has no access; as if music is somehow able to give him its content, to act as a "prosthesis" for his missing frontal lobes, for the brief time that he actually sings.[14]

---

13 This is not strictly true—Mr. S. did show anger, fear, or occasionally amusement, if he himself were directly involved. Thus, it was, rather, a lack of empathy he showed, a lack of concern for (or imagination of) the feelings of others. He lacked "secondary" but not "primary" emotions and in this way resembled the patients with prefrontal lobe damage described by Antonio Damasio:

> "These patients cannot generate emotions relative to the images conjured up by certain categories of situation and stimuli, and thus cannot have the ensuing feeling. ... Those same prefrontal patients can have primary emotions, however ... they would show fear if someone screamed unexpectedly right behind them, or if their houses shook in an earthquake." (*Descartes' Error*, 1994)

14 But what is the "content" of music? And how can it help the frontal-lobe patient to conjure up emotion-charged images, when an inability to do so forms the core of his disorder? One has the feeling, watching Mr. S. respond to music and sing, that music is somehow acting directly, giving him its mood, its mode, its "will" in a way that owes nothing to image or representation. This mysterious direct power is precisely what Schopenhauer speaks of in *The World as Will and Representation*:

> "...music, since it passes over the Ideas, is also quite independent of the phenomenal world, positively ignores it, and, to a certain extent, could still exist even if there were no world at all, which cannot be said of the other arts. Thus music is as *immediate* an objectification and copy of the whole *will* as the world itself is, indeed as the Ideas are. ... For this reason the effect of music is so very much more powerful and penetrating than is that of the other arts, for these others speak only of the shadow, but music of the essence (v. i., p. 257)."

The modulating and transforming power of music may also be very striking in people with autism who, for the most part, are so cut off from emotional experience or expression. I have observed this recently, with a young autistic savant, Stephen W., in England. Stephen has a repertoire of social reactions based on rote learning, and not on feeling, and a remarkable talent for visual analysis and drawing—this, too, unassociated with much feeling. The only time I have known him to show (and, one must infer, experience) vivid feelings in the years that I have known him has been in the context of music. He is able to sing and dance with real life and feeling with free, "normal," appropriate voice and movements. The external manifestations of his autism (the stilted postures, the averted gaze, the tics) all vanish, and he seems, for the duration of the song or dance, entirely normal. It seems, when he is singing, that he may be able to access a whole range of emotions and states of mind that are, for the most part, unreachable by him.

The "core" disorder in autism is very profound: there seems to be a radical impairment of the powers of imagination, communication and play; in a sense of one's own self and of others' selves in what is often called "theory of mind." This seems to based on a very complex and not yet wholly delineated neurological disorder—and yet, briefly, all this can be transcended with the performance of music, allowing at least the appearance of a normal emotional and imaginative identity.

This I have found the most astonishing, the least explicable, of all. With Harry, Greg, or patients with dementia, music acts as a mnemonic or reminder, recalling the person to his former self, forming a lifeline through apathy, amnesia, or dementia. This is wonderful to see but not too surprising, for it is akin to the effect of music on us all. But in the case of Stephen, music seems not so much a reminder, as a conferer, a creator of self, something that makes possible (if only briefly) that immensely complex neural and psychic integration that underlies the organization of a self.[15]

The question is whether this newly created or borrowed identity can achieve any sort of stability or permanence, or whether it must vanish along with the music. Indeed, this is the central question in relation to all music therapy—but particularly tantalizing, poignant, in the case of autism, for it may provide the first, or only, glimpse of a possible identity. There is some evidence, at least, that over and above its immediate effects, music can sometimes inaugurate a whole integrative process in the autistic, and lead to permanent changes in their lives. This was first shown by Nordhoff and Robbins (it is discussed in their book, and illustrated in their remarkable film, "The Music Child"), and is being explored in various centers about the world.

---

15 But it may be that in all of us, and not just the autistic, music not only has the power to evoke lost or forgotten or inaccessible parts of ourselves but to impose its own identity and "will" on us and in a manner that may sometimes be disquieting and unwelcome. Tolstoy was immensely sensitive to the power of music and passionately resentful, at times, that it could exert such power on him. His great short story "Kreutzer Sonata" describes how rage at the irresistable power of music finally provokes the protagonist to murder.

I have recently heard about a music therapy project with six autistic people in Birmingham, England, who not only respond to music "in a direct and utterly refreshing way," but have been showing, with the duration of the project, "a marked improvement in social skills and general adjustment"—an improvement not achievable, previously, in any other way. Ginger Clarkson, a music therapist at Yale, has been observing similar effects, while working closely with individuals who are autistic people.

Although there has been some observational and experimental work on the responses of animals to music, it is in human behavior that music plays such a wide role, and in the human nervous system, seemingly, that it has a such a wide representation. One must suspect the latter not only from the observations on the powers of music therapy we have considered, but from the relatively high incidence of musical "disturbances" of various sorts. Musical hallucinations are far commoner than visual hallucinations, for instance, and though they are sometimes associated with deafness (deafferentation), inner ear disease, tinnitus, toxic disturbances (salicylism) or epilepsy, they may also occur in the absence of any demonstrable pathology, especially in older people.[16] There seems even to be a sort of normal "reminiscence" or "recycling" of early musical memories—songs especially—in the aging (but otherwise intact) brain. Our brains, indeed, seem peculiarly given to a tenacious holding and replaying of musical stimuli; this is why tunes may be "catchy," and repeat themselves endlessly, sometimes maddeningly, in the mind.

The relatively high incidence of musical memories—either alone, or as part of a remembered or fantasied "scene"—was especially noted by Wilder Penfield in his study of the "experiential seizures" which may occur in temporal lobe epilepsy: the epileptic music, in such patients, may be elicited when the brain is exposed at surgery, with electrical stimulation of the epileptogenic cortical points. Music may itself precipitate seizures in some patients—so called musicogenic epilepsy (one such patient, described in the literature, was a music critic who was forced by his increasing intolerance of music to change his profession). But music may also have a strong *anti*epileptic (and also antimigrainous) effect.[17]

---

16 This became very clear to me when an essay of mine on musical epilepsy ("Reminiscence," Sacks 1986) was excerpted in the nationally syndicated "Dear Abby" column. I received hundreds of letters from people with intrusive musical hallucinations, most without obvious organic causes. Whether such hallucinated music, if it occurs in the brain of a composer, may aid creativity has been discussed both with regard to Schumann and Shostakovich. Schumann (so Peter Ostwald suggests, in *Schumann, Music and Madness*) may have been subject to an involuntary musical imagery of near-uncontrollable intensity—associated with manic-depressive or schizo-affective disorder, and perhaps some ear disorder too—but was able to use this for his own creative purposes until his tragic breakdown in the 1850s, when he found himself besieged by "demonic music" and "the music of angels," and, finally, by a single endlessly prolonged, intolerably loud tone. There was considerable discussion, ten years ago, about Shostakovich's "secret," following an article in the *New York Times*. It was suggested that he had a mobile shell fragment in the temporal horn of his left ventricle, and that "each time he leaned his head to one side he could hear music ... melodies—different each time—that he then made use of when composing."

Rhythm is central to all music; without it, music would cease to be music. But rhythm can be played out with the hands, the feet, the head, the mouth, the voice, the whole body. Its representation does not depend on any single motor modality. Thus, as Merlin Donald observes, rhythmic ability is "*supra*modal...evidence of a central mimetic controller that ... can interrelate the activities of these modalities in an incredibly rapid and subtle manner." Virtually all human cultures, Donald points out, use rhythm expressively, and its mimetic power survives many types of brain injury, both right- and left-hemisphere. Mimetic ability, Donald argues, is a peculiarly human achievement, beyond the powers of any prehuman primates—self-sufficient, but also a stage on the way to symbolic reasoning and language. These considerations may be very relevant to the basic powers of music and music therapy.

We have been seeing for several decades, above all in this present "Decade of the Brain," a huge and accelerating understanding of disease and health at the molecular level, the genetic, and the neuronal level—at the "micro" level. There has been far less research, and there is far less understanding, regarding the determinants of behavior and neural integration at the global or "macro" level. (Every level, of course, interacts with every other level.) And yet such determination is no less real, and no less important, than everything that goes on at the micro level. It is at a macro level, clearly, that music works.

But the higher levels of neural organization and integration are only beginning to be explored. We lack adequate concepts at this time (although we may have at least the beginnings of a coherent global theory of the brain in Gerald Edelman's theory of neuronal group selection) and, equally, we lack the appropriate experimental methods and tools. We cannot look at the activity of a million or ten million neurons simultaneously, and the orchestration (in Edelman's terms) of all their reentrant interactions and global mappings. And yet this is precisely what we may need to do if we are to understand human perception and consciousness and language, and, not least, the nature of the musical response.

---

[17] Both these pathogenic and therapeutic effects may be reflected at the level of the individual neuron. Thus Creutzfeldt, recording neuronal activity in conscious patients while exposing them to classical music, folk music, or drumming, found a suppression of discharge rate—a "calming" effect—most evident with classical music (above all with Mozart), and increased and synchronized ("entrained") discharges with drumming and loud rock music. Similar responses were observed in cats.

The responses of animals to music is a matter, as yet, more in the realm of anecdote than proof. The famous Lippizaner horses in Vienna are readily trained to respond to music, but this does not mean that horses naturally respond to it. There is a parrot in the movie "The Ladykillers" who bobs up and down on its perch in time to the strains of a Boccherini minuet; it is not clear to me whether this is the result of training or not. I have heard that goldfish may swim in time with Strauss waltzes and that mice can be conditioned to distinguish Bach from Mozart, but neither of these stories is adequately confirmed. Paderewski, in his memoirs (pp. 89–91) writes of a spider that could apparently distinguish thirds from sixths and would come down from the ceiling to the piano whenever he played Chopin studies in thirds, only to decamp ("sometimes, I used to think, quite angrily," Paderewski adds) when he switched to studies in sixths. One must wonder, too, about the possible responses of the human fetus to music—all sorts of vibrations, musical and otherwise, are readily transmitted to it, perhaps even amplified by the amniotic fluid.

References

Aldridge, David. "Rhthym Man" in A. Seligman and J. Hilkevich, editors. *Don't Think About Monkeys: Extraordinary Stories Written by People with Tourette's Syndrome.* Duarte, CA: Hope Press, 1992.

Clive, Geoffrey, editor. *The Philosophy of Nietzsche.* New York: NAL, 1965. (see esp. section on music, pp. 258–310.)

Creutzfeldt, Otto. Neuronal activity in the human lateral temporal lobe: activity during music, *Expt. Brain Research.* (1988) 77:490–498.

Critchley, MacDonald and Henson, R.A. editors. *Music and the Brain: Studies in the Neurology of Music.* London: Heinemann, 1977

Damasio, Antonio R. *Descartes' Error: Emotion, Reason, and the Human Brain.* New York: Grosset/Putnam, 1994.

Edelman, Gerald. *Bright Air, Brilliant Fire.* New York: Basic Books, 1992.

Luria, A.R. *The Working Brain*, tr. Basil Haigh, London: Allen Lane, 1973.

Nordhoff, Paul and Robbins, Clive. *Therapy in Music for Handicapped Children*, London: Gollancz, 1985.

Ostwald, Peter. *Schumann, Music and Madness*, London: Gollancz, 1985.

Penfield, W. and Perot, P. The brain's record of visual and auditory experience: a final summary and discussion, *Brain*, (1963) 86:595–696.

Sacks, Oliver. *The Man who Mistook his Wife for a Hat.* New York: Harper Collins, 1986.

Sacks, Oliver. *Awakenings.* New York: HarperCollins, rev. ed. 1990.

Sacks, Oliver. The last hippie, in *An Anthropologist on Mars.* New York: Knopf, 1995

Sacks, Oliver. A new vision of the mind, *New York Review of Books*, April 8, 1993, pp. 42–49.

Sacks, Oliver. *A Leg to Stand On.* New York: HarperCollins, rev. ed. 1994.

Schopenhauer, Arthur. *The World as Will and Representation*, tr. E.F.J. Payne. New York: Dover, 1958. (see esp. "On the Metaphysics of Music," vol. ii, chap. 39)

A delightful general book, covering every aspect of the human disposition to music, is *Music and the Mind*, by the psychiatrist Anthony Storr (New York: Free Press, 1992). This contains an excellent chapter on the clinical uses of music and music therapy.

CHAPTER 2

MUSIC AND MEMORY: ACCESSING RESIDUAL FUNCTION

Concetta M. Tomaino, ACMT-BC

Memory. What is the function of memory? How much do we actually remember? Can our bodies remember what our minds cannot? For many years now, I have been fascinated by the concept of memory function and of its resiliency despite severe neurologic injury and, most especially, by the power of music to retrieve otherwise lost functions.

My interest began as a student when I worked at a special program for handicapped children. It was my first exposure to the therapeutic use of music. How some of these children who had very limited function could participate and be so normalized within the context of a music therapy session amazed me. Later, I had the opportunity to do an internship in a small nursing home in Brooklyn. I was asked to start a music program for the most severely impaired residents who were immobile or restless and unaware of their surroundings. Most were not aware of their own identities. Their response to music took me by surprise. Not only did they immediately become animated, moving in time to the rhythm, but some who had not spoken for months started to sing. Anyone who works with persons with severe dementia can attest to the suddenness of these responses. What was happening? It appeared that there were elements, inherent in the music itself, that provided a gateway to lost function. The next year, 1980, I began my work at Beth Abraham Hospital. Within two days, I met Oliver Sacks, who provided the mentorship I needed to increase my understanding of neurologic function.

Those of you who have heard me before know that I'm very much interested in long-term memory and neurologic functioning. When someone with amnesia or dementia has lost his or her memory, it is amazing to observe how a specific piece of music will help that person recall information. Obviously they have cognitive damage. They can't process or sequence things the way other people can. There is something about the music and the songs themselves that embody a part of their personality and a part of their history that comes to life when they hear "their" music. Despite severe cortical damage, they still respond on the personal level; and this is what really fascinates me and has fascinated Oliver Sacks as well.

There are two elements of music, rhythm and melody (by melody I am referring to the power of a familiar melody to trigger emotional responses and long-term memory retrieval), that seem to have the greatest impact on function and also have parallel neurologic correlates. In the book *Music and the Brain*, by Critchley and Henson, N. Wertheim states:

> "There is no meaning to a rhythm without a message, and the impact upon the listener depends on this message carried by the rhythm, or else lent to it by the listener himself. We know this particular area of the brain stem, the reticular system, is concerned with a regulation of the cortical electrical rhythms ... there are abundant connections between the reticular formation and the auditory pathways. It may be that the rhythmical component of the auditory input has an impact on the whole cerebral cortex and also on large subcortical areas, via the extensive connections of the reticular formation with all these regions."[1]

The auditory nerve has an almost immediate connection to the midbrain. This area also called the limbic system is considered to be the emotional center of the brain (see Figure 1).

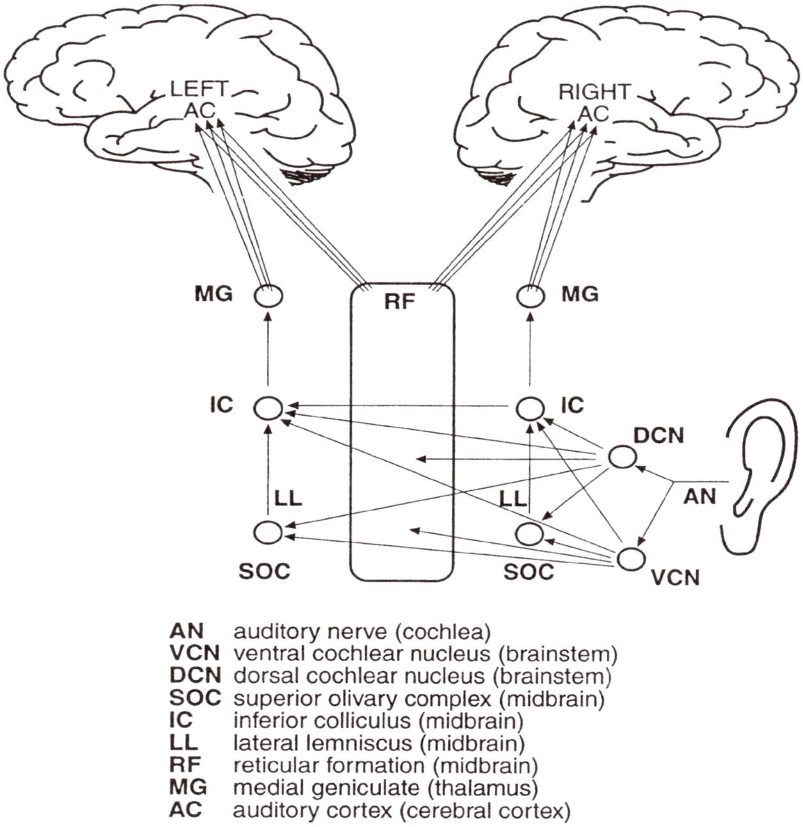

Figure 1. Schematic drawing of the ascending auditory pathways from *Handbook of Music Psychology, 2nd edition*. Donald A. Hodges, editor. © Copyright 1996 IMR Press. Used by permission.

You may observe this "limbic connection" clinically when you play a song for a patient and he or she immediately becomes alert, smiles, or cries. You observe a very personal and emotional response before you hear the song identified. First the rhythm helps focus the person's attention, then the melodic line/harmonies stimulate an emotional response.

Schopenhauer speaks of music as being different from the other arts, because it is not a copy of ideas but is more powerful and penetrating.[2] A single song can encapsulate an entire period of one's life, and hearing it can restore the essence of that reality.

In helping define Music Medicine, Koepchen et al. provides the following scheme of the bidirectional relations between the components of brain function and those of music, illustrating the role of neurovegetative rhythmicity in the framework of these relations (see Figure 2).[3] Neurovegetative rhythms include such functions as homeostasis, heartrate, bloodflow, and respiration.

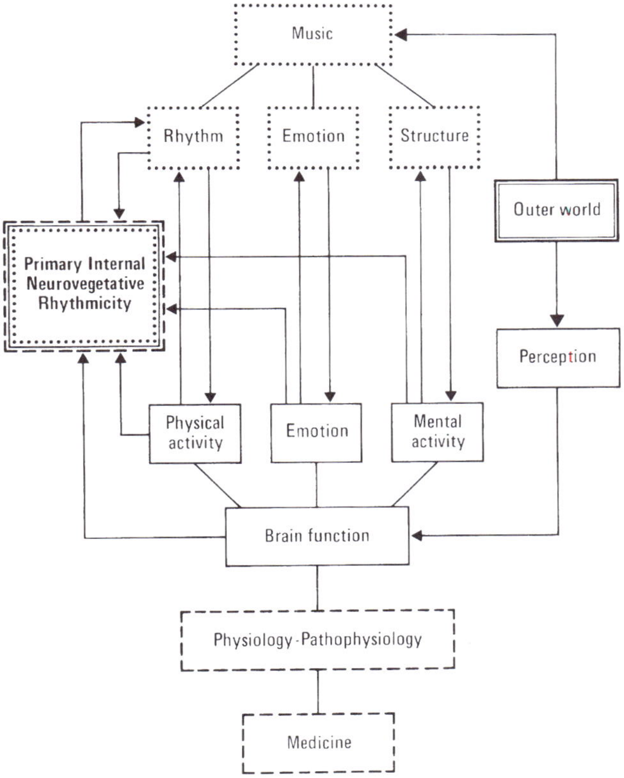

Figure 2. from *MusicMedicine*, Ralph Spintge and Roland Droh, editors. © Copyright 1992 MMB Music, Inc.

Looking again at the diagram of the ascending auditory pathways (see Figure 1), you immediately see that sound is represented bilaterally. Even if a person were deaf in one ear, he or she would still process music in both cortical hemispheres. This bilateral representation, with strong connections to the reticular formation, may allow for music to be processed even in persons with cortical damage. The auditory signal may be processed through an alternate network, thus circumventing the damaged area. This may also explain why we as clinicians observe responses that can not be rationalized or objectified through scientific means. Only when the technology improves may we start to know what neural processes are taking place.

There are different types of memory as well. Larry Squire (1987), a prominent figure in memory theory research, describes two contrasting types of memory that utilize different neurologic processes.[4] *Declarative memory* is more cognitive, fast, and adapted for one-trial learning. It permits storage of exact memories of a specific nature, such as time or place. It includes that which can be declared or brought to mind as an image. *Procedural memory* is slowly acquired over time from rehearsing a skill or task. It is developed and maintained through the specific network created in the formation of that skill. Procedural memory includes motor skills, cognitive skills, and simple classical conditioning. What is interesting is that most of the responses to music we observe clinically can be attributed to procedural memory. People who used to dance can still dance, even though they cannot walk as well anymore. Those who have lost their memories for other events in their lives can recall music quite well. It is possible that emotionally charged events are recalled throughout one's life and that recalling firmly establishes the memory. If a song is associated with the event, then just a single hearing of that song can stimulate the essence of that memory.

The first clinical case that I would like to describe to you is of a woman admitted following a hip fracture and evidence of dementia. She presented herself as somewhat agitated, although she would be calmed if she were given personal attention. She had persevervative speech and said "lady, lady, lady ..." continuously. When she heard a familiar song, she would sing it word for word. If she did not recall the lyrics, she would sing the melody on "la," with no trace of perseveration. The following videotape illustrates her responses within the music therapy sessions. It starts with her sitting motionless with a drumstick on her lapboard. As the music starts, and she slowly becomes engaged; she picks up the drumstick, and follows the rhythm very slowly. She progressively moves the stick from her lapboard to the drum at her side. Once she hits the drum and starts playing, she remains engaged throughout that session. She could be engaged for 20 to 40 minutes, doing just the drumming alone. Once she is connected in the rhythm, I introduce an Italian song that she knows. She sings the complete lyrics without a hint of perseveration. Several sessions later, during a "good morning song" that one of the other patients created, Ms. A. sings along "Good Morning, good morning to me" (pointing to herself as she says the words). She is now integrating the meaning of the lyrics. A few seconds later she stops singing and says, "I'm tickled". "Tickled?" I ask. "By the music!" She exclaims and opens out her arms. This was the only coherent sentence she had produced in quite some time. Ms. A., like many persons with dementia, could not connect to the world around her, yet the capacity for involvement was there. She needed the music to organize and to call to her as a person. This provided a means to engage her on a very personal level.

Ms. S. had a diagnosis of leuco-encephalopathy. She did not speak, except to say her name was Sally. She was easily frightened, at least when she was first admitted. Despite her confusion, she could walk the length of the hallway without incident. This was quite remarkable, given that she seemed to have a visual agnosia and could not make sense of objects in her environment. She could perhaps figure out where a table was, but it was only by accident. She would walk into it, touch it, and only then realize it was a table. She would then reach over to find a chair. Since she did not speak, it was difficult to discern her level of cognitive functioning. She obviously couldn't be tested, because she couldn't answer any of the questionnaires. She was alert, watchful, and did seem to have some emotional responses to staff.

One day, during a music therapy session on Ms. S's unit, I came to realize how aware Ms. S. was. I was playing some songs from the 1920s and 1930s. Ms. S. walked in and out of the group, paced up and down the hall, each time remaining a little longer in the group. At one point, I heard a beautiful, strong voice singing all the lyrics. I turned, thinking it was a staff member, only to see Sally dancing and singing with the music. I did not stop the music and played one song after the other. As long as the music continued, Sally continued, fully engaged, almost entranced. I had a chance to talk with her sister later on that week to find out if there were anything about Sally I should know and why this music was so familiar to her. Her sister said that Sally used to play the piano all the time. Many of her favorite songs were the same tunes I had played during the session. Her sister also stated that Sally had not touched the piano in years and stopped singing just prior to her illness. Her sister was surprised that Sally could make a coherent sound, let alone sing lyrics. Music became part of Sally's daily routine. The physician's assistant on the unit was an excellent singer. Together we designed short phrases that could be used to communicate to Sally. Soon the other staff joined in. Sally started to sing responses to the staff, and she became less agitated and withdrawn. Within a few months, she was able to sit down and be part of the music therapy session for the duration of the group.

When we speak of memory function, we often think of factual memory. However, we also possess postural schema for physical movements. These are very well preserved and can be called to through music. Manny was a new admission to this facility. In addition to physical limitations, he had dementia. He thought that he was in a VA Hospital at the end of World War II, recovering from an enemy bullet. He was here for long-term care and spent his day seated at the dining room table. He could walk with assistance but had poor balance.

He would often stumble, shuffle along, and tire easily. When I played some upbeat dance tempo melodies, however, he would jump out of his chair and dance around the room. I called his family to find out something about him, because he just stepped up and started dancing and could dance an hour or two. His daughter said that he used to dance at the Savoy Club; in fact, he was part of a group that used to dance there quite a bit. His dancing was such a part of him that this ability was better preserved than walking. His dancing became a means of increased physical activity that eventually aided his physical recovery, and he was discharged to his daughter's home. Roger Sessions speaks of rhythm and movement as being integral to our nature. Sessions states,

> "the basic ingredient of music is not so much sound as movement ... I would even go a step farther and say that music is significant for us as human beings principally because it embodies movement of a specifically human type that goes to the roots of our being and takes shape in the inner gestures which [that] embody our deepest and most intimate responses".[5]

The idea of separate movement schema is a fascinating one; the possibility of which is clearly demonstrated with Manny. For most of us, movement is a natural activity; something that we do without much thought. To a person who has lost physical functioning, due to head trauma or stroke, the concept of what it feels like to move becomes all-encompassing. Yet, if this person is stimulated to move spontaneously, he can often accomplish a range of activity that would otherwise be impossible. The potential for movement may be there, but the ability to self-initiate movement is lacking. We have even observed cases of persons with severe contractures who can relax and allow passive range of motion when a strong rhythmic musical cue is provided.

In *Philosophy of the Body* Meleau-Ponty states, "A movement is learned, when the body has understood it; that is, when it has incorporated it into its 'world;' and to move one's body is to aim at things through it; it is to allow oneself to respond to their call, that is made upon it independently of any representation. Motility, then, is not, as it were, a handmaid of consciousness, transporting the body to that point in space of which we have formed representation beforehand. In order that we may be able to move our body toward the object, the object must first exist for it, our body must not belong to the realm of the 'in-itself' ".[6] So, even to become part of the environment is to interact or participate with something outside of oneself. It must first be internalized and become a part of the person. And that happens with both movement and music—given the right rhythm and the right melody.

Not too long ago we had a visit by a reporter from *Reader's Digest* who was interested in learning more about music therapy. I introduced him to a middle-aged woman with whom I was working. She was here for short-term rehabilitation but showed early signs of dementia. She clearly described how music kept her connected. While I played, and she sang, an older resident with Alzheimer's disease who was pacing the hallway heard the music and came over to us. As I played, his posture changed. He reached out his arm to the other patient and took her by the hand, and they danced around the hallway. For that moment, he was a different person. The staff who were watching were incredibly moved by this, and, when the music stopped, the reporter asked Mr. A. how he liked the music. Mr. A., who was not very articulate, said, "It gets you right here," pointing to his heart. He then walked off to the hallway.

Sam is a man in his late 60's who is recovering from a recent stroke. He was on physical therapy and was considered a "guarded walker"—he could walk independently with a quad cane, but he wasn't steady enough to walk outside, as he would have difficulty negotiating the uneven pavement. He was referred to music therapy in hopes that he could improve his proprioception and his ability to sway his body. Since he had left-side weakness, his left leg never came off the floor. He was able to tell me about his background, and how, as a teenager, he used to go dancing every week at the gym. He had not really danced since then. The physical therapist tested Sam's gait, and I found some music with a tempo that matched the pace of his stride. The music was familiar to him, and he felt comfortable walking to the tempo. As he became more confident of his movements, he began to add dance steps, sliding his feet or clicking his heels. As the sessions progressed, he became more inventive in his movements; and, within several weeks of meeting twice a week, he began lifting his left foot off the floor. He was not aware of this but stated that he was able to feel the tempo in his leg and thought that he actually was able to feel the floor with his left foot. He had previously mentioned that one of the most frustrating things for him was to go to the entertainment programs here and have his right foot tap away, while his left foot remained immobile. Now he was regaining sensation in that side. In the following video example you will see Sam "dancing" to Nat King Cole's "Walking My Baby Back Home". It is evident that he is able to lift his foot off the floor and that all his steps are synchronized to the music. When the music stops and he is asked to walk, his steps become less regular and he drags his left foot. We worked together for two months, and he was also working with a physical therapist who was trying to get Sam to think about the song and the rhythm when he began losing his stride. Sam was soon discharged and moved to an apartment in the community.

Dr. Michael Thaut, a music therapist and researcher at the University of Colorado, has documented the effects of rhythmic cueing on gait.[7] I have also observed clinically that a strong rhythmic beat can induce movement and help maintain walking in patients with impaired gait. Although rhythm is enough to cue gait, the more one can internalize the music the more likely there will be a carry-over outside of the therapy session. Sam stated that when he felt his leg dragging he would just sing the song to himself, and his leg would start to behave again.

This is a similar phenomena to what happens in Parkinson's disease, showing the effect that music and rhythm has on aiding the initiation of movement. I was working with a young man in the community with Parkinson's disease. He stated that he needed something to get him "unstuck" during the day.

We explored a whole inventory of music and different types of rhythms that would work for him. He found that it wasn't music with strong down beats, like march tempo or swing-time tempo, that would work for him, but rather music that had an anticipatory beat like African drumming, that helped him get organized and anticipate his next step. It was the anticipation that he needed to stimulate movement.

I put together a series of tapes for him to use with his Walkman, whenever he needed to go out. When he felt that he was going to get stuck he just switched on the tape and the music carried him to his destination. He also used imagery and internalization of the feeling of the rhythm to help him when he did not have the tapes. In contrast, he had difficulty relaxing at times, especially in the evening. Another tape was designed to provide music which gradually became slower, eventually lulling him to sleep.

These are just a few cases that illustrate how music can help one gain access to residual cognitive and physical functioning. To summarize, let me go back to how music is used for persons with dementia, and then also how music is used for people with gait problems.

Rhythm is very important. It is used to stimulate attention and spontaneous responses, to coordinate movement, and to engage and hold the person through the intervention. Even a person with severe dementia and/or attention deficits can improve his attention level, over time, with rhythmic stimulation which can engage him spontaneously.

Songs play an essential role. To stimulate recognition memory, the more emotionally charged the song is, the more likely a person will respond. Even when they have deteriorated and can no longer make appropriate connections to the music, there is a "sense of knowing", a "sense of familiarity" that can provide a feeling of comfort and security to one who has lost all connections to the outside world. As with Sally, the woman with leukoencephalopathy, this ability of music to provide a feeling of security can aid in the transition to a new and unfamiliar environment.

Responses to music can serve as a *diagnostic tool.* What does the response look like? Has there been a change over time? Does the response change with different rhythms or melodies? Is the voice expressive or monotone? I remember one woman who was able to sing many songs with excellent voice quality, but several months after admission I noticed that the quality of her singing had changed. The melodic contour was gone, although the rhythmic character of the song was intact. I pointed this out to the attending physician. The unit staff had not noticed a change, as she was still able to speak. The physician ordered some tests and discovered that she had suffered a slight stroke in the right temporal region.

In using music to enhance gait and other physical functions, there are several factors to remember. What is the person's comfortable walking pace? Request this assessment from the physical therapist. What is the person's musical history? Select music with tempo corresponding to the appropriate pace.

Select music of interest to the person, as there will be a better chance of carry-over of relearned skills. Live music is preferable, as the tempo can be adjusted as needed. However, pretaped music can be used if the patient requires some supervision/contact guarding while ambulating, or if the music is to be used by the patient independent of the music therapy session.

The potential for the use of music as a therapeutic tool in neurologic rehabilitation is only beginning to be understood. The clinical evidence has been documented and discussed. It is hoped that as technological advances occur, especially in the area of neuroimaging, we will be able to understand fully the multiple processes of memory, the complexity of neural networks, and mostly, how music connects to essential neurologic function.

References

Calvin, William H. *The Cerebral Symphony.* New York: Bantam Books, 1990.

Critchley, MacDonald, and Henson, R.A. *Music and the Brain.* London: William Heinemann Medical Books, 1977.

Davis, John Booth. *The Psychology of Music.* Stanford: StanfordUniversity Press, 1978.

Hodges, Donald A. editor. *Handbook of Music Psychology*, 2nd edition. San Antonio, Texas: Institute for Music Research Press, University of Texas at San Antonio, 1996.

LeDoux, Joseph, and Hirst, William.. *Mind and Brain.* New York: Cambridge University Press, 1986.

Spicker, Stuart, editor. *The Philosophy of the Body*, Chicago: Quadrangle Books, 1970.

Spintge, Ralph, and Droh, Roland. *MusicMedicine.* St. Louis: MMB Music, 1992.

Squire, Larry. *Memory and Brain.* New York: Oxford University Press, 1987.

Squire, Larry, and Butters, Nelson. *Neuropsychology of Memory.* New York: Guilford Press, 1984.

Storr, Aanthony. *Music and the Mind.* New York: The Free Press, 1992.

Thaut, Michael H. and McIntosh, G.C. "Effects of Rhythmic Auditory Cueing on Stride and EMG patterns in Normal Gait", *Journal of Neurologic Rehabilitation*, 1992, Vol. 6, pp. 185–190.

1. N. Wertheim, in Critchley and Henson. *Music and the Brain*, London: William Heinemann Medical Books, 1997, p. 293.
2. Schopenhauer, Arthur. *The World and Will as Representation.* Cited in Anthony Storr. *Music and the Mind.* New York: The Free Press, 1992.
3. Koepchen, H.P., Droh, R., Spingte, R., Abel, H., Klussendorf, D., and, Koralewski, E. "Physiological Rhythmicity and Music in Medicine" in Spintge and Droh. *MusicMedicine.* St. Louis: MMB Music, 1992, p. 45.
4. Squire, Larry. *Memory and Brain.* New York: Oxford University Press, 1987, p. 162.
5. Sessions, Roger. *The Musical Experience of Composer, Performer and Listener.* in Anthony Storr. *Music and the Mind.* New York: The Free Press, 1992.
6. Meleau-Ponty. "Spatiality and Motility". In Stuart Spicker, editor *The Philosophy of the Body.* Chicago: Quadrangle Books, 1970, p. 260.
7. Thaut, Michael H., & McIntosh, G.C. Effects of Rhythmic Auditory Cueing on Stride and EMG patterns in Normal Gait. *Journal of Neurologic Rehabilitation*, 1992, Vol. 6, pp. 185–190.

CHAPTER 3

MUSIC FOR PERSONS WITH DEMENTIA AND THEIR CAREGIVERS

Alicia Ann Clair, Ph.D., RMT-BC

Introduction

Patient Characteristics

This presentation is based on research and clinical work conducted by Alicia Ann Clair, Ph.D., RMT-BC, through the Recreation Service at Colmery-O'Neil Veterans Affairs Medical Center in Topeka, Kansas. The work began with efforts to determine the types of programming that would be viable in a population of persons diagnosed with dementia, including those with probable Alzheimer's type, who had progressed in their disease until they were severely debilitated. These persons, who were veterans, were also patients in the medical center. They were at high risk for personal security and safety. They could no longer be maintained in their homes, due to wandering, agitation and other behaviors that posed severe problems to their family caregivers. Consequently, they were admitted to a secured unit at the Veterans Affairs Medical Center where they could receive 24-hour care and supervision.

These patients were characterized with short attention spans, and little or no orientation to time, person or place. They often were so out of touch with their surroundings that they bumped into each other, tripped over one another, or tried to sit in chairs already occupied. In their confusion, they were often involved in incidents of physical combativeness with one another and with staff. Most remembered their wives who came to visit, at least during the early months of hospitalization, but they often did not know their children or even the family pet that was once so dear to them. Many had hallucinations and/or delusions and most were isolated from others through their confusion.

These persons could no longer engage in usual purposeful activities alone or with others. They often required help eating and some did not eat at all unless fed by staff or family members, usually their spouses. Most required assistance with toileting and some were incontinent. Many of the patients on the unit required comprehensive care and supervision with all activities of daily living.

All but two of the twenty-eight patients on the unit were male, since the medical center serves veterans; and the majority of United States veterans are men. They came from a very large and primarily rural area that made the distance from home great for some. Consequently, visits from family and friends were difficult and sometimes impossible, but many of the men had spouses who continued to visit throughout their hospitalization on the unit. Some wives relocated their homes to live nearby.

The mission of the hospital unit was to provide care for these patients in their late stages of dementia, until the disease progressed to the point that patients were no longer at risk for safety and needed only the nursing services provided in a residential care home. At that point, determined by team review in consultation with the family or guardian, appropriate placement was made into the community.

Spouse and Family Caregiver Characteristics

Family members and spouses brought their patients to the medical center out of sheer desperation. They had no resources left, either personal or physical, with which to continue to cope with primary caregiving. They had suffered extreme stressors as they cared for a person who continued to debilitate. Many of these caregivers had to terminate their employment and were in financial devastation; and, often these caregivers had manifested their own physical illnesses to the point that they were directed by the physicians to discontinue their caregiving, or they would themselves require hospitalization. Many caregivers had become hypertensive. Some had developed cancer and other serious illnesses. Many of them were either overweight or underweight, as meal preparation became impossible; and they had to grab food on the run. They had no time for themselves and no opportunities to meet their own needs. They were hypervigilant at all times, knowing that loosing sight of their loved one for even a few seconds could result in peril or even tragedy.

As the caregiving became more intense throughout the disease process, these caregivers became more and more isolated from their friends and family. The length of the disease process, which can range from eight to twelve years and even longer, had far outlived the abilities of most friends to "stick by." They no longer had the companionship or emotional intimacy their spouses or parents had provided through the years, and other family members often found it quite difficult to tolerate persons in their conditions of dementia.

Without support, these spouses and family caregivers suffered through tremendous losses entirely alone; and, when they could no longer cope, they brought their family member in for care. Most caregivers had a clear understanding of the disease diagnosis when they arrived; but, for many, the full impact of the prognosis had not yet hit. Some hospitalized their family members, so they could have respite themselves, only to realize and admit, after several weeks, that they could not deal with the fact that their loved ones were never going to recuperate from their disease and that they would become progressively more debilitated until they died. Some of these caregivers and their families left their patients at the medical center and did not come to visit.

Some spouses prepared themselves for a lengthy, terminal illness. They moved into residences near the hospital, gathered all the resources they could and hung on; but, whatever the circumstance, these spouses were hurting emotionally, and their families were hurting also.

Support groups were available to all family caregivers to provide education, information, emotional support, and any other assistance that was necessary. In addition to the support group these caregivers and their families were always welcomed in the medical center unit. They had access to nursing and other support staff, were included in unit activities, and participated in their family members' team reviews. Their input into their loved ones' care plans was considered essential to care and treatment.

As these caregivers became more involved in unit activities, that staff became a source of support and even became their family. These caregivers, whose lives had been fraught with anxiety and fear for years, experienced great relief with their relative's hospitalization. As the patients adjusted to the routine and settled into the predictable, secure structure of the unit, these caregivers made efforts to regain their strength. Without the burden of full-time, primary care, the family had opportunities to recover. Caregiving spouses continued, however, in their social isolation, especially if they had relocated their homes. They were neither widowed nor married in the traditional sense and did not fit readily into society. They were no longer a part of a viable couple and were not included in couple activities. It took great courage for them to survive, even though they no longer had primary caregiving responsibilities. With all of this, they had even more losses to come. Among these were the eventual discharges of their spouses into residential care, which resulted in the termination of relationships with the medical center staff who had become family, the financial devastation due to extended medical care, the end of retirement dreams and plans for the future, and their own aging and potential physical disabilities.

Music Therapy Programs and Research

Initial Music Therapy Programming and Outcome

An early survey of the unit and initial conferences with nursing staff members revealed that there was little or no programming for patients, due to their extremely short attention spans and apparent lack of interest. The staff was very invested in providing the best possible care and believed that involvement in activities other than daily unit routine was essential. There was just no information concerning program implementation with patients who were so severely regressed. This staff eagerly welcomed music therapy services to the unit and was supportive in every way.

Music therapists attempted a wide variety of strategies. These included, among others, movement to music, massage, and singing and playing rhythm instruments. It was soon revealed that patients participated most often in rhythm playing and tended to prefer vibrotactile to nonvibrotactile responses. These observations were supported in several small sample research studies (Clair and Bernstein 1990a; Clair and Bernstein 1990b; Clair, 1991). Additional research showed this vibrotactile response was not associated with tactile stimulation provided by tape recordings of varying music media (Clair and Bernstein, 1993). Also, it became clear that not only those with music background and not only those who were indicated by nursing staff as most compliant could participate successfully (Clair, 1990).

Music seemed to quiet and calm patients, even when they were distressed, but this observation is based only on anecdotal information and not on empirical research. In fact, one study revealed no statistically significant differences in incidents of agitated behaviors under conditions of stimulative music, sedative music and no music (Clair and Bernstein, 1994.) Although the results of this study showed no statistical significance among the conditions studied, the influence of music on the behaviors of those with dementia bears further investigation.

Further observation of persons hospitalized with late stage dementia showed that these patients tended to discontinue their singing as their diseases progressed, but they continued to participate readily in rhythm activities (Clair and Bernstein, 1990a.) They also sat for periods of 30 to 45 minutes without restraint while participating in music therapy sessions (Clair and Bernstein, 1990b.)

Observations showed that these patients did not tolerate massage well, and that they intended to draw away from physical contact unless it was provided as a cue for rhythmic movement with music. These patients continued to move in rhythm until they reached very late stages in the disease process and ambulatory patients danced, particularly if they had prior experience dancing.

Music Therapy with Family/Spouse Caregivers

Caregivers were incorporated into music therapy whenever they were present on the unit during scheduled sessions. As they participated, they shared their amazement that their loved one could participate in purposeful activities as a member of a group. They indicated at times that they saw flashes of their care receivers as they used to be and that participation in music provided opportunities for them to interact together with their care receivers in nonverbal ways. It was music therapy that some way tapped residual skills and abilities and provided the means for successful and meaningful experiences. For this, family caregivers expressed deep appreciation.

It became apparent that music therapy programming could be designed to incorporate the family caregivers into sessions, and these caregivers were asked to participate in music therapy at the medical center on a regular basis. Following their participation, the caregivers provided verbal feedback that resulted in the development of a music therapy practice protocol that was subsequently pilot tested in the community.

The pilot-tested protocol was conducted once weekly for eight weeks with four couples in which one person in the couple had a diagnosis of probable Alzheimer's disease but had not progressed to the point of hospitalization. The goal was to provide the opportunity for couples to leave their isolation, brought on by care and behavioral management requirements in the home, and again to relate socially as a couple with others in a like circumstance. The protocol, which began with lunch at a restaurant, was followed by a 30-minute music therapy session that included singing, ballroom dancing and rhythm participation, primarily drumming (Clair, Tebb and Bernstein, 1993.) There were strong indications from hospitalized and nonhospitalized couples that music therapy was viable, effectitious and desirable. It provided opportunities for couples to work together and to interact socially and purposefully with one another and with other couples. Music provided the means to achieve social integration to some degree for all participants.

Couples Protocol Outcomes

Opportunities to sing were provided to couples both in the medical center and in the community pilot test group. There were differences, however, in the abilities to recall and sing songs. The hospitalized patients did not recall words and did not acknowledge recalling melodies to songs that were popular in their young adult years. If they sang at all, and some of them did not, they sang familiar folk songs of their young school age years. These included such selections as "Home on the Range," "I've Been Workin' on the Railroad" and others. Even with these selections, participants required frequent prompting through verbal reminders to participate.

In contrast, persons still in the community were eager singers and participated well in using song books with a wide range of song selections. They sang consistently with only an initial cue from the lead music therapist. Some individuals even sang harmony and expressed verbally their pleasure with the opportunities to sing.

Singing was followed by ballroom dancing, which was successful for all ambulatory individuals regardless of the severity of their dementia. The dancing was first attempted at the medical center with one couple who had not danced in over 20 years. Following the session in which they danced, the patient's wife said that she was so delighted that she had the opportunity. It was the first time that her husband had held her in his arms for three years, and she had missed him terribly. They were no longer able to have verbal conversations, they had lost their opportunities to share emotional intimacy, and the dancing recovered one way in which they could be close.

Dancing in the pilot program was greeted with enthusiasm by three couples who had danced together earlier in their lives, but one couple had never danced. Although this couple attempted to dance in the first two sessions, the husband's physical limitations made it uncomfortable; and they discontinued participation in the dancing segment of the sessions.

Other couples were excellent dancers; and although they had not danced in years, their recovery was quick; and the smiles of delight were continuous. After three of the six sessions, one caregiving wife said that her husband had asked her to dance at home in the kitchen one day while she was making lunch. She stopped her preparations and they danced to a tune on the radio. She was delighted, and dancing in the kitchen became a regular activity for them at home.

Drumming made up the last segment of each session. It was successful for couples with one hospitalized member and for couples who did not yet require hospitalization. It seemed that drumming was a quick success for all participants. Responses were made immediately upon placing the drum in the individual's hands. These responses were rhythmic and musically sensitive.

Most patients played in a form in which a clear beginning and ending were evident. With great consistency, participants entrained together, beating in time with one another. This phenomenon occurred spontaneously with even the most regressed patients.

Rhythm Characteristics

It is clear from the observations made over the last several years that active rhythm participation is likely for success with persons who are in the late stages of dementia. It is important to note that when individuals deteriorate to a certain point in late stage dementia, they will not likely respond by playing rhythm instruments such as drums. It may be possible that they will make other responses to music, such as opening their eyes or turning their heads when musical stimuli are present, but much is yet unknown concerning responses to music in persons with very late stage dementia.

It seems that rhythm is basic to humans at all stages of life, and it provides organization and structure in the environment. Rhythm is predictable in nature and, therefore, provides a secure pattern into which individuals can enter. It is through such structure and predictability that persons who have little internal organization can fit in conjoint efforts with others. It provides opportunities to "belong with others", an aspect of their lives that has been lost through the confusion and devastation of their dementias.

A subsequent research effort sponsored by the Rhythm for Life Project, funded by the Tides Foundation, further supported positive participation in rhythm (Clair, Bernstien & Johnson, 1995.) Outcomes of this study demonstrate that individuals retain capacities to 1) participate in call/response patterns, 2) imitate specific rhythm patterns, and 3) perform spontaneous rhythm patterns. Their participation is active and carries on, generally, without pervasive verbal or physical cues but is dependent on structure provided by a trained music therapist. Individuals' musical backgrounds, their presence or absence, seem to influence their abilities to imitate rhythm patterns. Those individuals who studied music as youngsters seem more capable of imitating progressively more complex rhythm patterns than those who did not study music.

Most individuals, although they had no prior experience with drumming, indicate their enjoyment with it either through facial expressions or verbalizations, or both. Family and residential care home staff are very supportive of individuals' participation and verbally indicate their delight, and initially their surprise, in successful participations. Some care home staff have said that they noticed residents' apparent relaxation after participating in the rhythm sessions. This is anecdotal and may be a phenomenon associated with expectation.

Summary

Clinical research has begun to demonstrate that music therapy is viable and effectitious for persons diagnosed with dementia and their caregivers. There is evidence that persons can participate successfully, alone or with others, in purposeful activities using music, even into the late stages of their disease process. There is also evidence that caregivers can use music as a way to interact and maintain some elements of the relationships they have shared through the years with their loved ones. These relationships are essential to caregivers and care receivers as they go through the disease process together.

There is very little that is known about the therapeutic applications and functional uses of music, but there is a beginning. To develop further the knowledge in this area, it is important to continue to document with research the clinical music therapy practices appropriate for persons with dementia and their family caregivers.

References

Clair, A. A. The need for supervision to manage behavior in the elderly care home resident and the implications for music therapy practice. *Music Therapy Perspectives, 8,* 72–75, 1990.

Clair, A. A. Rhythmic responses in elderly and their implications for music therapy practice. *Journal of the International Association of Music for the Handicapped, 6,* 3–11, 1991.

Clair, A. A. and Bernstein, B. A comparison of singing, vibrotactile and nonvibrotactile instrumental playing responses in severely regressed persons with dementia of the Alzheimer's type. *Journal of Music Therapy, 27,* 119–125, 1990a.

Clair, A. A. and Bernstein, B. A preliminary study of music therapy programming for severely regressed persons with Alzheimer's type dementia. *Journal of Applied Gerontology, 9,* 299–311, 1990b.

Clair, A. A. and Bernstein, B. The preference for vibrotactile versus auditory stimuli in severely regressed persons with dementia of the Alzheimer's type compared with dementia due to ethanol abuse. *Music Therapy Perspectives,* 11, 24-27, 1993.

Clair, A. A. and Bernstein, B. The effect of no music, stimulative music and sedative music on agitated behaviors in persons with severe dementia. *Activities, Adaptations and Aging, 19,* 61–70, 1994.

Clair, A. A., Bernstein, B., and Johnson, G. Rhythmic characteristics in persons diagnosed with dementia, including those with probable Alzheimer's type. *Journal of Music Therapy, 33,* 234–247, 1995.

Clair, A. A., Tebb, S. and Bernstein B. The effects of a socialization and music therapy intervention on self-esteem and loneliness in spouse caregivers of those diagnosed with dementia of the Alzheimer's type: A pilot study. *The American Journal of Alzheimer's Care and Related Disorders and Research, January/February,* 24–32, 1993.

CHAPTER 4

PARAVERBAL PSYCHOMOTOR TECHNIQUES IN NEUROLOGIC HABILITATION AND REHABILITATION

Helen Mandel Grob, M.M. RMT-BC, CPvT.

In addressing the subject of the symposium, the author feels it necessary to refine the focus on "rehabilitation" to include "habilitation." Differentiation of these terms is contingent on the prognosis of specific conditions and consequently will determine the input and approach utilized. Rehabilitation implies restoration. This may be pursued in specific traumas/insults to a once intact and functioning CNS such as CVAs, other closed head injuries, spinal cord injuries and so on. In these instances, we may see the victim regain lost abilities that may reflect in specific or all social/affective, communicative, cognitive and motor domains. Here, habilitation connotes the ability or means by which one may cope within a specific handicapping situation or condition. Among these are degenerative diseases where impairment is progressive and not restorative, such as: Alzheimer's disease, Parkinson's disease, AIDS, Pick's disease, and Huntington's disease.

One neurological condition that is unique in that it may be considered to fall into both categories is autism. It is nondegenerative but manifests progressive, severe, and bizarre behaviors that peak around ages 6–7 and then level off.

Those autistics identified as falling into both categories are those who reveal a degree of abstractive ability and are responsive to facilitated communication (FC).[5,2] In these cases, we may be considered to be "rehabilitating," in that we are "restoring" or gaining access to an ability that was untapped, and "habilitating," in that a means is being provided to cope with the condition via a channel to communicate. The ability to communicate may reflect in all domains.

For this symposium, Huntington's disease (HD) was selected because of its unique characteristics requiring a global approach[1, 4, 6, 17-19, 21, 25] and because of the possibility that some of the responses to the techniques used[17, 18] may be applicable to other neurologically involved conditions and lead to further speculation and channels for exploration. These may include autism with regard to FC, panic anxiety attacks described by Grandin[7, 8, 9] and other congenital CNS impairment exhibiting SBs and SIBs. The latter of which has been documented.[12]

To describe the approach utilized, it is necessary to differentiate recreational activities, which has its merit, from therapeutic services. In providing therapeutic services, the therapist should be knowledgeable in the responses of the components and characteristics of music in social/affective, communicative, cognitive and motor domains, all of which relate to the CNS.

Consequently, the individual or combined components and characteristics of music are utilized for diagnostic assessments to establish goals, objectives and methodologies and to serve as a possible vehicle to achieve them.

Obviously, the music therapist need not be a musician of virtuoso or performance calibre, nor use music primarily for its æsthetic sense, but for its effect and responses involving the aforementioned domains. The professional training of the music therapist has been detailed and described.[15]

In addressing the topic of the symposium, the focus is on the CNS and its responses to specific aspects of music, which has been described in the literature.[3, 10–18, 22, 23, 26, 28] The approach that encompasses the aforementioned are paraverbal techniques based on paraverbal therapy. Paraverbal therapy was developed and practiced within a psychiatric framework.[20] Paraverbal techniques maintain the psychiatric framework that has been modified and expanded to include a neuropsychological and developmental framework as well. The description of paraverbal techniques and its clinical application to a broad spectrum of progressive and static disorders and pathologies has been established, described and documented.[10–18, 28]

In Huntington's disease, the developmental aspect of paraverbal techniques assumes importance in diagnosis in that symptoms appearing prior to 15 years of age exhibit different characteristics than the symptoms of an adult. Victims have been reported to have been misdiagnosed.[19, 25, 18] The developmental aspect also comes into play in assessing deterioration that varies in rate and domain.[17]

In servicing clients with Huntington's disease, the need for psychiatric grounding associated with paraverbal techniques becomes evident. While dementia is ascribed to Huntington's disease victims,[1,6] this has not been evident until end stages of the disease and then not present in all cases.[17,18] Victims are particularly aware of their deterioration. Consequently, some develop coping mechanisms to maintain their autonomy and ego. The degree to which these coping mechanisms are manifest is contingent on the basic personality of the victim.[17,18] Knowledge of each patient's behavior and competency in behavioral strategies is required by the therapist to address each individual.

Within the neurological framework of Huntington's disease, peripheral nerve fibers effecting messages transmitted to muscles and to the CNS appear intact, as opposed to aberrant neuronal messages transmitted in the reverse, causing choreiform and rigid movements.

Paraverbal techniques using rhythmic, cyclic, and sensory (visual, kinesthetic, tactile, auditory, vestibular, and proprioceptive) input, including dual dependent rhythmic motor tasks to these intact peripheral fibers, have revealed inhibition of choreiform movements and increased fluidity in rigid movements.[17,18]

Such input is congruent to that sought by some autistics[7,8 9,13] and others with congenital brain impairment where SBs and SIBs are manifest. Similar application of paraverbal techniques to those exhibiting the aforementioned have yielded positive results in extinguishing exceptional behaviors.[12,13] The approach appears to be effective in interrupting or rechanneling aberrant neuronal transmitter discharge.

There are those with intact and functioning CNSs who have suffered CVAs. Some result in specific aphasias where there is right hemispheric functioning and prosody remains intact. It has been reported that MIT, which employs paraverbal techniques, has been successful in rehabilitation.[28]

The aforementioned and documented responses to music utilizing paraverbal/psychomotor techniques may yield further channels for exploration and application in rehabilitation and habilitation to an expanded spectrum of neurological involvement.

References

1. Bayles, K. "Linguistic communication disorders of dementing diseases." Paper presented to the International Neuropsychological Society Conference, San Antonio, Texas, 1991.
2. Biklen, D. Communication unbound: autism and praxis. *Harvard Educational Review.* Vol. 60, No. 3:291–314, 1990.
3. Bjorkvold, J. "Child culture and music education." Report presented at the International Conference of Biology of Music Making: music and child development and personal contact. University of Colorado, Denver, 1987.
4. Brothers, C. Huntington's chorea in Victoria and Tasmania. *Journal of Neural Science* 1:405–20, 1964.
5. Crossley, R. "Communication training involving facilitated communication." Paper presented to the Australian Association of Special Education Annual Conference. Canberra, Australia, 1990.
6. Folstein, S. *Huntington's Disease—a disorder of families.* Baltimore: John Hopkins University Press, 1989.
7. Grandin, T., Scariano, M. *Emergence—labeled autistic.* Novato: Arena Press, 1986.
8. Grandin, T. "An inside view of autism." Paper presented at the 43rd Annual National Association for Music Therapy Conference, personal communication, St. Louis, Misssouri, 1992.
9. Grandin, T. "Autism." Paper presented at Autistic Society of America, New York, 1993.
10. Grob, H. "The use of music in differential diagnosis." Paper presented at the 25th Annual National Conference of the National Association for Music Therapy, Philadelphia, October 22–26, 1974.
11. Grob, H. "Music Therapy." in Valletutti, P.J. and Christopolos, F., editors. *Preventing Physical and Mental Disabilities: Interdisciplinary Programs.* Baltimore: University Park Press, 1979, pp. 197-210.
12. Grob, H. "Paraverbal techniques with focus on stereotypic and self-injurious behaviors." Paper presented at National Conference of the Association for the Severely Handicapped, New York, 1981.
13. Grob, H. "Music and paraverbal techniques with autistic children." Paper presented at Regional Conference—Autism: New Directions, Adelphi University, Garden City, New York, 1982.
14. Grob, H. "The use of music and paraverbal techniques in the diagnosis and treatment of specific learning disabilities." Paper presented at the 37th Annual Conference of The National Association for Music Therapy, Chicago, Illinois, 1986.
15. Grob, H. "Clinical Training Programs in Music Therapy: The International State of the Art" in *Proceedings of Internation Society for Music Education Commission on Music Therapy and Music in Special Education*, Melbourne, Australia, 1988.
16. Grob, H. "The use of music and paraverbal techniques with children afflicted with AIDS" in *Proceedings of Canadian Music Therapy Association*, 1990.

17. Grob, H. "Music Therapy." Presented as faculty at First International Interdisciplinary Training Course: Caring for persons with Huntington's Disease—New York Medical College, Huntington's Disease Society of America and Foundation for Care and Cure of Huntington's Disease, 1991.

18. Grob, H. "Use of music and paraverbal techniques in degenerative diseases" in *Current Research in Arts Medicine*. Chicago: A Cappella Books, 1993.

19. Hayden, M. *Huntington's chorea*. New York: Springer-Verlag, 1981.

20. Heimlich, E. Paraverbal techniques in the therapy of childhood communication disorders. *International Journal Child Psychotherapy*, 1:65–82, 1971.

21. Jackson, H. *Selected Writings of John Hughlings Jackson*. London, Hoddler and Staughton, 1931.

22. Kohut, H. Observation on the psychological functions of music. *Journal of the American Psychoanalysis Association*, 5:389–407, 1957.

23. Mayer, W. Live composers dead audiences. *New York Times Magazine*, 12:12–42, 1975.

24. Mittleman, B. Mobility in infants, children and adults. *Psychoanalytic Study of Children* 9:142–177, 1954.

25. Myers R., Martin, J. Huntington's Disease. *Neurology*. 2:365–72, 1982.

26. Payne, E. Elephant talk. *National Geographic*, August, 1989.

27. Rourke, B. "Syndrome of nonverbal learning disabilities: manifestations in neurological disease, disorder and dysfunction." Paper presented at Annual Conference of the New York Neuropsychology Group, 1991.

28. Sparks, R., Helm, N. and Albert, M. Aphasia Rehabilitation Resulting from Melodic Information Therapy. *Cortex*, 10, 303–316, 1974.

CHAPTER 5

DIGITAL MUSIC TECHNOLOGY IN MUSIC THERAPY PRACTICE

Joseph Nagler, DA, CMT

People and Technology

This is an exciting time in human history. Our world is experiencing profound and wondrous changes. The world, as we understand it, appears to be getting smaller, while it becomes more complex on a daily basis. As we unravel more secrets, new and more enigmatic challenges arise. New understandings of our world are also creating new challenges for our study. Many of these opportunities have become evident through investigations and applications of digital technologies.

Digital technologies, once the province of an elite few, are now infused into many aspects of our contemporary society. Digital technologies now appear on our desks, laps, wrists, belts, and even in our pockets. Information is now more accessible and ever present. To paraphrase Wordsworth (1888) : "The digital world is too much with us, late and soon." We browse, e-mail, and share information with ever increasing ease and clarity. We now accept digital data as a given.

Everyone and anyone can be a publisher of information. The emergence of this phenomena has democratized the process of being heard and seen to a broad community of individuals. This democratization allows us to enhance our humanness through the communication of our ideas. Yet, the aesthetic experiences we share depend largely upon our ability to ascribe to a set of norms and values that surround the experience. We dialogue through very carefully crafted means of interaction; we are our experiences (Nagler, 1995.)

Communicating these experiences is a relatively new phenomena. We, as a society, have arrived at new fertile ground, in which a new order of interaction is emerging. The digitizing of our daily interactions into data is increasing in practice and importance. Digital data have permeated our homes, work, and, ultimately, our lives. Digital data have manifested themselves in many ways into our lives. We conduct commerce, exchange ideas, and create representations of entities, all through digital data. We have grown increasingly more dependent upon digital data to communicate efficiently.

It appears that our cultural understanding has accepted the perception that we function in collective aesthetic activities as limited by our functional abilities. Dictating these functional abilities are our innate skills, education and training, along with our abilities to communicate ideas to one another. If this axiom is indeed valid, then a great many ideas will remain unexpressed until a cogent medium of expression avails itself to the person. But is our acceptance of digital technologies an accurate reflection of our cultural Zeitgeist?

The very use of technology can be an alienating, asocial behavior. As we expand our "cyber" world, we may sacrifice important aspects of our real world. This is too new an entity for us to begin to understand the long term affects of our interactions. Users can dedicate an inordinate amount of time and energy to their machines; machines that are emotionless and, at times, unpredictable. Our technologies are clumsy, inconvenient, "hardly something with which you might wish to curl up with in bed" (Negroponte, 1995, pg. 11.) While nascent in form and frustrating to operate, computers have changed daily life for many. These machines can represent a dramatic shift in the order of our societies.

Still, not all of these changes are positive. We conform to the operational limitations of our machines. We contort our bodies to interact with these machines. We anthropomorphize our computers and assail their quirky characters. We even form allegiances to one computer operating system over another, as if it were some form of a religious entity. Still, technology is becoming ubiquitous.

Technology for People with Disabilities

Perhaps nowhere is technology more ubiquitous than in the lives of people with physical disabilities. People with neurological, congenital, or other incapacitating infirmities have benefited immensely from the omnipresence of technology in our societies. Speech, communication, ambulation, mobility, activities of daily living and even tactile stimulation can all be enhanced digitally. Disability no longer equals exclusion. Necessity has created devices that enable, empower, and liberate many people with infirmities from the confines of their physical limitations. A cogent example of this is exemplified by what occurs when a person's functional disabilities preclude daily interaction. When a person experiences a marked inability to communicate with the world around her it diminishes and hampers the expression of her humanness. It also can effect her place in society and ultimately, the quality of her life. Technological solutions provide the medium for purposeful self-expression. In essence, technological innovations have aided the further assimilation of people with physical disabilities to mainstream society.

People with powerful minds but less able bodies have been liberated to a proper place in society. This shift is a testament to the persistence and perseverance of individuals with disabilities who are effecting these changes. Digital technologies have played a pivotal role as an agent of change for this group of people.

Music and Digital Music Technology

One area in which technology has emerged as a powerful entity is in enhancing the process in the creation of music. Never before has sound and music been more accessible. This is due, in part, to the emergence of new digital music technologies used to enjoy sound and music. Digital music technology has grown at a rapid pace in the past fifty years. The act of digitizing sound to a series of binary numbers has created a new genre for self-expression. People of varied musical and aesthetic training can create rich sonic tapestries. Many of these sonic possibilities were not possible even a decade ago.

The evolution of music technology in the latter part of this century has catapulted digital music technologies from the university lab to the home desktop. The advent of the Musical Instrument Digital Interface (MIDI) was the first step in the popularization of the "private" digital music technologies movement. The ability to capture Digital Audio on desktop systems, was the second step. The new availability of desktop multimedia via the Internet and internal operating system of desktop computers opens a new avenue for self-expression using digital music technologies.

The future holds the lateralization of emerging technologies to create expressive personal digital music technologies. Internet-based solutions that combine with more powerful computers allow individuals, regardless of physical functionality to create music in new and expressive ways.

Music Therapy

Music therapy is a therapeutic modality in which people create music in an attempt to achieve a better sense of health and well-being. Music therapy using digital music technology is often used with people who are in need of physical assistance to create music. When this type of intervention is employed in conjunction with a medical setting with people having neuro-muscular disorders, a primary role of the therapist is to aid in physically providing a voice for those who cannot share their own. Music therapy in medicine is defined as "the therapist uses musical experiences and the relationships that develop through them as a means of helping medical patients to gain greater control over their illness, treatment or convalescence." (Bruscia, 1989, pg. 130.)

Music therapy is a safe, effective and economical form of therapeutic intervention in a medical setting (Lee, Bejanni, & Nagler 1991.) In a medical setting, music therapy can be used to enhance cognitive abilities, increase physical abilities, increase communication abilities, enhance self-esteem and personal sense of self, and enhance ability to create art. (Nagler & Lee, 1985.)

The process of music therapy as it is practiced by this author is multifaceted. The primary focus of this therapeutic approach is participating in the process of creating music. While the end musical "products" are essential and vital to the therapeutic outcomes, they are not the primary reason for therapeutic interventions. Conversely, it is the self-awareness and discovery occurring from participation that is the primary function of music in therapy. The role of the therapist is to provide an atmosphere in which this therapeutic exploration can occur.

The process of music therapy embraces the act of creating music as an essential part of a therapeutic process. For many people, it is a large step toward the road to health. The aesthetic experience of music used in a therapeutic process has brought forth new and inventive ways for reaching people with neurological and neuromuscular impairments.

The use of music and, more specifically, music therapy to aid in the rehabilitation of neurological impairments is a relatively new discipline. Music therapy interventions can provide people new opportunities to transcend physical, emotional and cognitive barriers with immediacy and clarity. Music therapy can provide a vehicle for the expression of thoughts, feelings, and actions that may lay dormant and locked for many years. It appears that the combination of sound and the skills of a music therapist can have a positive influence on the rehabilitation process.

One researcher has attempted to define the elements of music that contribute to its healing power. In her discussion of music and healing, Bonny (1986) found that music contains five distinct characteristics that render it suitable for use in therapeutic work. These attributes are (1) Music is nonverbal, (2) Music evokes emotional responses, (3) Music evokes physiological responses, (4) Music stimulates symbolic representation, and (5) The sensory stimulation of music can create synesthesias of other senses.

In neurological rehabilitation, all five of these components of music play equally important roles in the patient's and therapist's relationships to music. The physiological responses have been studied in several settings. (Bailey, 1983, Bonny 1983, Skille, Wigram, & Weekes, 1989.) These studies have explored the physiological responses demonstrated by patients in response to various musical stimuli. Psychological responses of patients to treatment in music therapy were studied by Hodges, (1980) and Davies, (1978) with regard to the measurement and nature of musical behaviors. Additionally, the nonverbal and the symbolic uses of music were explored in the study of the use of Blissymbolics with cerebral palsied children. (Herman, 1985.)

Yet, little has been written about the use of music in the neurological rehabilitation process. Brescia & Opher (1993) have reported several recurring themes evidenced in the music therapy process. These themes include spirituality, sense of body image, sexuality, and issues related to the healing process. Additionally, the emotional life of patients as evidenced in the music therapy process and relationships to significant others was studied. Musical preferences as related to the music therapy process as evidenced in interactive song writing played an important role in this study.

Often, individuals with physical limitations cannot create music on traditional instruments intended primarily for musical performance by people without severe physical limitations. These traditional instruments are not malleable to each person's unique physical limits. Many people are excluded from the music-making process.

Music Therapy and Digital Music Technology with Neurologic Rehabilitation

Digital music technologies can augment functional abilities and replicate many aspects of human musical performance encountered by people with severe physical limitations. Through the use of digital musical instruments to create "networks" of sound-producing devices, a person can create the virtual "one-man band" with very gratifying results. Digital musical technology can be used to create new and different sounds that can redefine the music-making process.

The use of digital musical technology in clinical music therapy settings can be combined with a dynamic, patient-directed therapeutic method. This method includes the playing of precomposed songs and clinical improvisation to meet the patient's communicative, cognitive, emotional, and physiological needs. The instruments used in this therapeutic method are a hybrid of digital music technologies and traditional acoustic instruments. The music created as a part of this method can be both culturally and aesthetically congruent to the needs of many inner-city adolescents.

This article will now describe a research study involving digital music technology with neurologically impaired inner-city adolescents. This investigation was a collaborative effort between the New York City Board of Education and New York University Medical Center's Rusk Institute of Rehabilitation Medicine. The primary purpose of this inquiry was to study clinical music therapy interventions as they were applied in the treatment of neurological disorders. The therapeutic interventions took place over an eight-week period. During that time, the participants received music therapy treatment twice weekly. The participants of the study were adolescent males.

The findings reported in this article pertain to a singular case. While there were several participants in this study, one person was chosen to demonstrate both the interventions and the research and reporting methods employed in documenting the interventions. The participant profiled in this article is a sixteen-year-old African-American male with cerebral palsy. He is categorized as a spastic quadriplegic with mild learning disabilities.

The musical instruments employed in this process are instruments traditionally found in a clinical music therapy practice, combined with digital musical instruments. The category of traditional or acoustic musical instruments commonly include an upright piano, a guitar, drums, and a rich assortment of hand-held percussion instruments. The sound-making capabilities of these instruments are rich and varied.

In addition to the traditional instruments, digital musical instruments were employed extensively in this study. A computer equipped with MIDI sequencing software and a MIDI interface, along with a Drum MIDI controller, an upright piano, and several synthesizers were employed.

A Case Study

This case is reported as an illustration of the power of music and music therapy exacting a change in a person's way of being. Willie, the participant profiled, is a truly distinctive person. Unable to speak, walk, or use any of his extremities, Willie has navigated his world in unique and wonderful ways. To date, despite what was originally classified as a mild mental retardation and then later, learning disabilities, Willie has recorded a set of truly remarkable achievements. He is an author, a lecturer, a computer resource person, and now a musician. As the following construct demonstrates, Willie is a motivated person.

Qualitative research is emerging as a valid and reliable method of researching the process of music therapy (Wheeler, 1995.) The use of thematic analysis in the form of vignettes is an emerging trend in qualitative research (Lincoln & Guba, 1985.) The term "constructs" is often used to describe this technique (Bannister & Fransella, 1989.) The data are reconstructed by the researcher in order to attain clarity in the process of the data analysis. Constructs are "distilled from the data in as close a likeness as possible of the participant's mode of expression. The intention is to present in miniature the essence of what the researcher has seen and heard over time" (Ely, et al., 1992, p.154.) The following is a construct of the person profiled in the case study.

Construct: Willie

"Music—makes me whole, a lot better. You know it's like I was born to do this. I mean I've only been playing for a few weeks, and already I can pick out songs with this metal stick that's attached with Velcro to my forehead. It's really different that something comes so easily to me. Everything I have ever done has been a real struggle. From talking to people to getting around by myself. Life isn't easy when you can't speak or move your arms and legs. I get frustrated a lot. So, please don't judge me by my mechanical-sounding voice. I wish I could do more. It would help to get what I need. It would help me to stop people from doing things to me they know they shouldn't do.

But I can move my head. I can move it to do just about anything. I can bowl, play a tabletop hockey game, and, yes, I can make music all by myself. I can do it! I sit and watch and learn. I take in everything that's around me. Watch and learn, watch and learn. I really like computers. I'm very good at using one. I have a job working in a center that helps other people like me to use computers to do work.

I started out playing the blues. I followed Joe and played what he played. After a while, I started to play and Joe followed me. We talk to each other in the music. It's like I've finally found a way of talking that comes naturally.

I have a girlfriend. I really like her. Her favorite song is "The One" by Elton John. I learned this song to play it for her. It was easy. I had to learn to read music. I learned to read music quickly, even though I fake it sometimes. The song wasn't that easy to learn, but I can do it. You see, I can do it because music— makes me whole, a lot better."

Discussion

Willie has received music therapy treatment for eight weeks. He came into the initial session and requested to play a keyboard. Considering the severity of his neurological impairments, it appeared that this would be a difficult task for him to perform. Willie insisted that he had never done this before but he knew that he could accomplish it if given the chance. The process of getting Willie to interact with a music keyboard synthesizer was a difficult one. Physically, the layout of the piano keys are longer than his range of motion. To compensate for this, the keyboard was reconfigured to have pitches normally associated with the middle register of the keyboard digitally remapped to the upper register. This allowed for greater access to a wider range of musically expressive tones that were within his reach. Willie accessed the tones he played on the keyboard through a pointer stick worn over his head like a baseball cap. This limited Willie's range of musical expression. He quickly learned to compensate for this by learning to slide from one note to another to give the appearance of playing two notes simultaneously.

To build a musical vocabulary quickly, Willie and I began our therapeutic process by playing the blues together. We first sequenced a blues pattern using a software program known as Band In A Box (BIAB.) BIAB allows for entry of musical chord patterns by simply typing the letter associated with that chord on a computer keyboard. For example, Willie could enter a Bb dominant seventh chord by typing the symbol "Bb7." The software algorithmically assigned rhythmic and harmonic functions to the chord symbols based on the style of music selected. We chose the style of "Blues Shuffle." I provided Willie with a lead sheet of a C blues pattern and asked him to enter this into the BIAB program.

Willie entered this pattern quickly and, soon thereafter, we were listening to "Willie's Blues." To begin our process of learning to communicate with one another, I began to demonstrate different blues melodies based on the following scale:

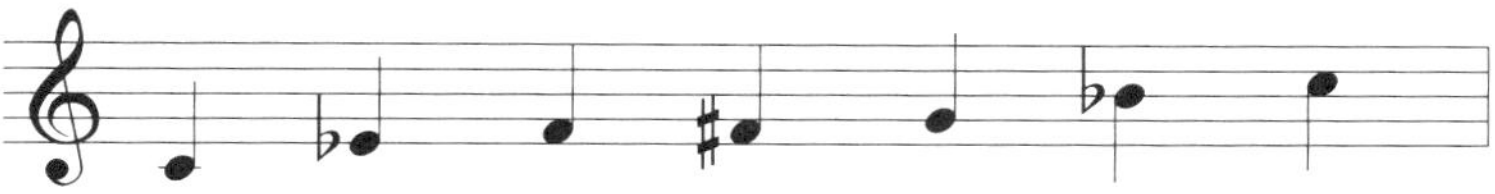

This led to musical coactivity between Willie and me. I would demonstrate a pattern, Willie imitated the part I played. We later reversed roles, and Willie initiated the pattern, and I imitated the idea and then embellished upon the original. Willie would then take my cue and further the musical conversation along. This led to a high level of interaction and discourse between us.

As our relationship grew, so did the sophistication of our music. After becoming more musically expressive in his blues playing, Willie began to seek more complex musical expression. In the course of four weeks, Willie progressed from never having played the keyboard to attempting to play Elton John's song "The One." His motivation to attempt playing this song was a combination of musical curiosity and the need to express his feelings toward his girlfriend.

For Willie, this was an opportunity to demonstrate in song what he previously was unable to express in actions, words, or his written work. Willie had found the voice he was looking for.

Conclusions

By his own account, the process of music therapy has been a rewarding and enriching experience for Willie. Music has aided Willie in creating a lifeway different from his normal routine. Music and, in part, music therapy have increased his level of freedom from his uncooperative physical being. Willie used the music as an enabler that assisted him in creating his own identity through both the metaphorical and tangible process of music making. Willie has grown from a passive listener of music to an active, creative participant in his own process of rehabilitation. Willie has reached a new level of growth and personal understanding regarding his therapeutic process.

In his brief experience in music therapy, Willie has found the means to express his innate musicality. His use of technology and adapted devices have aided in this self-expression. Additionally, his relationship to the timbres, music, and lyrics used in his therapeutic process have helped to bring to life his unique form of self-expression.

Despite severe developmental delays, both cognitive and physical, there was not only normal musical development but also extraordinary innate musical ability. Briggs, (1991) has profiled the concept of musical development as it relates to developmental milestones. In her model, Briggs presents four phases of musical development that parallel the psychological development of infants and toddlers. The four phases, Reflex, Intention, Control, and Integration, chronicle musical development from zero to sevetny-two months. Her model postulates that "music has a developmental schema, a schema that appears to be consistent in the literature and correlates with other major models of child development."

Willie, it appears, is an anomaly to this schema. His cognitive and physical development would not fit into this model. Briggs' scale presents her phases in terms of three categories or musical milestones. The first category, Auditory, demonstrates that Willie, indeed, has mastered all of the developmental skills. Yet, in terms of her categories of Vocal/Tonal and Rhythmic, Willie presents between the earliest of her phases, the Reflexive and the Intention phases. How can this disparity exist? I believe the answer is twofold. The first reason is due to the relationship that music plays in Willie's life as an emotional and aesthetic experience. Music was not a diversion; it was a living entity that Willie aspired to create. The second reason was Willie's ability to transcend his developmental deficits. He adapted not only the music to his needs but also the musical instruments themselves. Willie created music on musical instruments that were available and malleable to his musical and mechanical needs. The instruments functioned for him and not the converse. Willie was able to request different permutations of subtle yet significant changes that led to enabling him to use the instruments for his expression.

The primary intent of this article was to demonstrate that music therapy can serve as an integral component of a neurological rehabilitation process. Through the preceding case, I have attempted to demonstrate the power of music therapy to impact the lifeworld of a person with severe neurological impairments. The data presented within the context of the construct demonstrates Willie's experiences and the profound effect that this process availed to him. This data was validated by checking the construct with Willie for veracity and accuracy. It is important to note that while there are other methods of data reporting and analysis available, none of the existing methods will avail to the reader the richness of the therapeutic process nor the vitality of what transpired.

Alarming as it may be, many types of human interaction do not avail themselves to a numerical entity; reduction to statistical endpoints would serve to demonstrate that some changes did take place in the process. Yet, many of the other areas such as Willie's increases in self esteem, self expression and musical development would not have been reported with the same candor and richness. Clearly in this case, numerical apportionment of variables would have served little if no purpose in demonstrating what had transpired. Therefore, the use of the preceding construct is the clearest way of data presentation and interpretation. In closing, I would suggest that there is the need for substantial research in this area before any conclusions may be drawn as to the efficacy or the role of music therapy in rehabilitation. It is my hope that this article will serve to inspire further thought and study.

References

Bailey, L. M. The effects of live music versus tape recorded music on hospitalized cancer patients. *Music Therapy: Journal of the American Association for Music Therapy*, 3 (1), 1, 17–23, 1983.

Bannister, D. and Fransella, F. *Inquiring Man: the psychology of personal constructs.* London: Routledge, 1989.

Brescia, T. and Opher, K. An exploration recurring themes in the physical rehabilitation process as seen through songwriting and selection. In press, 1993.

Briggs, C. A. A model for understanding musical development. *Music Therapy: Journal of the American Association for Music Therapy*, 10 (1), 1–21, 1991.

Bruscia, K. (1989). *Defining Music Therapy.* Phoenixville, PA: Barcelona Press.

Bonny, H. L. Music listening for intensive coronary care units. *Music Therapy: Journal of the American Association for Music Therapy*, 3 (1), 4–16, 1983.

Bonny, H. L. Music and healing. *Music Therapy: Journal of the American Association for Music Therapy*, 6 A (1), 3–11, 1986.

Davies, J. B. *The Psychology of Music.* Stanford, CA: Stanford University Press, 1978.

Ely, E. with Anzul, M., Friedman, T., Garner, D. and McCormak-Steinmetz, A. *Doing Qualitative Research: Circles Within Circles.* Bristol, PA: The Falmer Press, 1991.

Herman, F. Music therapy for the young child with cerebral palsy who uses Blissymbols. *MusicTherapy: Journal of the American Association for Music Therapy*, 5 (1), 2, 28–36, 1985.

Hodges, D. A. *Handbook of Music Psychology.* Lawrence, KS: National Association for Music Therapy, 1980.

Lee, M. H., Bejanni, F. J., and Nagler, J. C. United States Senate Subcommittee on Aging: Forever Young with Music Therapy. One hundred and second Congress S. Hrg. 102.545 Serial No. 10, 102–9, 1991.

Lincoln, Y. & Guba, E. *Naturalistic Inquiry.* Beverly Hills, CA: Sage, 1985.

Nagler, J. C. and Lee, M. *Music Rehabilitation and Human Well Being.* St. Louis, MO: MMB Music, 1985.

Nagler, J. C. "A qualitative study of children in crisis: Interventions through music therapy and digital music technology." Unpublished doctoral dissertation, New York: New York University, 1993.

Nagler, J. C. Towards the aesthetic lifeworld. *Music Therapy: Journal of the American Association for Music Therapy*, 13 (1), 75–92, 1995.

Negroponte, N. *Being Digital.* New York: A. Knopf, 1995.

Skille, O., Wigram, T., & Weekes, L. Vibroacoustic Therapy: The therapeutic effect of low frequency sound on specific physical disorders and disabilities. *Journal of British Music Therapy*, 3 (2) 13–17, 1989.

Wheeler, B., editor. *Music Therapy Research.* Phoenixville, PA: Barcelona Press, 1995.

Wordsworth, W. *The Complete Poetical Works* ... With an introduction by John Morley. London: Macmillan and Co., 1888.

CHAPTER 6

Introducing "SOUNDBEAM"

Michael Hillman

Soundbeam is a MIDI controller that translates physical movement within space to musical sound. It sends out an ultrasonic beam, similar to radar, that detects the presence and range of any object that enters its area and converts this to MIDI data. It is small, safe, lightweight, well built and easy to operate.

In the two years I have used Soundbeam, I have found it to be a most versatile MIDI controller for children with various handicaps. In its most simple state, attached to a synthesizer, it allows children or adults who cannot make music with any other instrument to play the synthesizer in ways limited only by their imagination and musical sensitivity. Combined with a computer, it becomes a very powerful musical tool giving the user the capability to perform on many different levels or to compose music electronically.

Soundbeam has ten different settings or modes that allow for different scales, pitch variations or expressive capabilities. Each of these modes responds in different ways depending on the synthesizer attached to Soundbeam; but no matter what synthesizer is being used, one can obtain many interesting and beautiful musical effects. It would obviously seem that more expensive synthesizers would offer more possibilities, but even inexpensive models work well with Soundbeam and sometimes offer effects that are difficult to do with more expensive synthesizers. Yet, in a complete MIDI lab outfitted with a computer and a sophisticated sequencing program, the possibilities are endless.

I work with students ranging in age from five to nineteen years. Although over half live at the hospital, many go home nightly to various neighborhoods in the metropolitan New York area. These children have a wide range of physical and developmental needs resulting from many different causes, and each child has a different response to music in general and Soundbeam in particular. I find Soundbeam works best when I work with individual students, because our students arrive to class grouped by age, rather than abilities, and often are not as successful in a group setting. To help alleviate this problem, I have many types of music controllers, and I encourage the students to play together as a group whenever possible. Soundbeam is another means to this end.

I have used the Soundbeam with a computer for two years; and, during this time I have discovered the possibility of using it as a play along instrument and a tool for composition. One such way of doing this is to set Soundbeam to a single shot mode and set up the sequencing program into a loop; then, as the student records, the notes return over a set time. Eventually, the student is accompanying him- or herself. I also set my program up so the timbres are constantly being changed, which helps stimulate interest.

To use the Soundbeam with a prerecorded sequence, I set the computer up to play a scale into Soundbeam, which allows it to remember the scale when set on mode ten. The sequence then continues with an accompaniment pattern that fits my prerecorded scale. This saves time since all that remains is to turn Soundbeam on in mode ten and start the sequence. Soundbeam is then ready to play with the sequence.

Another possibility, if your sequencing program is able, is to have Soundbeam control other musical parameters, such as timbre, tempo, volume, or any other parameter your sequencing program can control. This can be done by creating a scale of pitches that the sequencing program reads as instructions for change.

If you own a commercial synthesizer that has auto-accompaniment patterns, you may try the following. Set the span so that the lower notes of the beam are in the bass section of the synthesizer. These notes will then trigger the chord changes in your auto-accompaniment mode. The type of synthesizer you use with Soundbeam will make a big difference in how you use it. Time and research should be spent in selecting a synthesizer, and it does not necessarily have to be an expensive model.

On a personal level, as a performer, I have found Soundbeam to be an interesting method of self-accompaniment. I set up a sequence with my computer, set Soundbeam to an appropriate mode, and accompany myself as I play trumpet.

To assess how effective a resource Soundbeam is, the manufacturer, EMS, would like you to consider the following:

Will it encourage body awareness?
Will it build confidence about movement?
Will it extend movement?
Will it help develop fine motor control?
Will it help the student explore cause and effect?
Will it encourage listening, attention and discrimination?
Will is stimulate imagination?
Will it encourage improvisation?
Will it build communication skills?
Will the student make music?
Will it foster a sense of achievement?
Will the student have fun?

Students of all ages and abilities respond to Soundbeam, and Soundbeam can be a valuable tool for anyone teaching movement of any kind, be it dance or physical therapy or self-awareness. It is a wonderful motivational tool to teach extension, fine motor control, body awareness or any physical movement. It is also a great attention grabber and a wonderful way for students to explore cause and effect and to stimulate awareness of sound as a structure. I highly recommend it as a tool for any therapist needing such a motivator. I have also discovered that a physical handicap makes little difference. If a student is musically sensitive, he or she will respond to Soundbeam with creativity and curiosity. If not, he or she will need time to develop the sensitivities to use Soundbeam as a musical instrument and not as a toy. In either case, it is a valuable musical tool that allows people who have never had access to traditional musical instruments an avenue for musical communication that is legitimate, expressive, and creative and allows them to participate in musical activities previously denied them.

Postscript:

It has been three years since I have left Blythedale, and I know that EMS has made several improvements in Soundbeam. I have learned that it is now controllable by computer and responds to MIDI program changes. I am sure that these improvements make Soundbeam an even more valuable tool for musical creativity and performance.

Reference

Silverman, M. *The Soundbeam Project, USA*. Bronx, NY: M. Silverman.